TEXTBOOK FOR DIALYSIS TECHNICIANS

TEXTBOOK FOR DIALYSIS TECHNICIANS

As per the Latest Guidelines and Syllabus

Editors

Narinder Pal Singh
MD FACP FRCP (Edin) FASN ISHF FISN FAMS FICP MBA
Academic Consultant Nephrology
Max Super Speciality Hospital
Saket, New Delhi, India
Dean Research (Volunteer)
Eternal University, Baru Sahib
Himachal Pradesh, India

Vineet Behera
MD DM FACP FASN FICP PGDTGC
Consultant Nephrologist
INHS Kalyani
Visakhapatnam, Andhra Pradesh, India

Foreword

Vivekanand Jha

Prologue

Vijay Kher

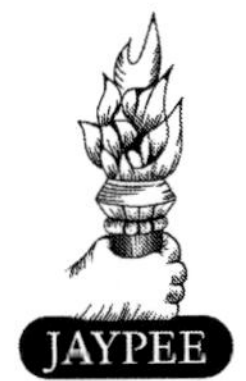

JAYPEE BROTHERS MEDICAL PUBLISHERS
The Health Sciences Publisher
New Delhi | London

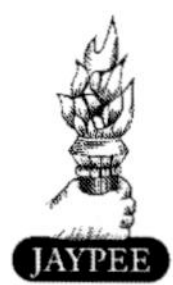

Jaypee Brothers Medical Publishers (P) Ltd

Headquarters
EMCA House, 23/23-B Ansari Road,
Daryaganj New Delhi 110 002, India
Landline: +91-11-23272143,
+91-11-23272703
+91-11-23282021, +91-11-23245672
e-mail: jaypee@jaypeebrothers.com

Corporate Office
4838/24, Ansari Road,
Daryaganj New Delhi 110 002, India
Phone: +91-11-43574357
Fax: +91-11-43574314
e-mail: jaypee@jaypeebrothers.com

Overseas Office
JP Medical Ltd.
83, Victoria Street, London
SW1H 0HW (UK)
Phone: +44-20 3170 8910
e-mail: info@jpmedpub.com

EU GPSR Authorised Representative
Logos Europe, 9 rue Nicolas Poussin
17000, La Rochelle, France
Phone: +33 (0) 6 67 93 73 78
e-mail: contact@logoseurope.eu

Website: www.jaypeebrothers.com
Website: www.jaypeedigital.com

Textbook for Dialysis Technicians
First Edition: 2024
Reprint: 2026
ISBN: 978-93-5696-585-0
Printed at: Samrat Offset Pvt. Ltd.

Contributors

Amit Katyal
Consultant Nephrologist
INHS Asvini
Mumbai, Maharashtra, India

Amra Ahsan
Associate Professor, Behavioural Sciences
Shree Guru Gobind Singh Tricentenary University
Gurugram, Haryana, India

Anil Kumar Bhalla
Senior Consultant and Chairman
Department of Nephrology
Sir Ganga Ram Hospital, New Delhi, India

Anish Kumar Gupta
Consultant Research, Faculty of
Medicine and Health Sciences
SGT University, Gurugram, Haryana, India

Arpita Roy Chowdhury
Professor and Head, Department of Nephrology
North Bengal Medical College and Hospital
Darjeeling, West Bengal, India

Arun Kumar S
Assistant Professor, Department of Nephrology
All India Institute of Medical Sciences
New Delhi, India

Aruna Acharya
Associate Professor and HOD, Nephrology
SCB Medical College and Hospital
Cuttack, Odisha, India

Asheesh Kumar
Assistant Professor, Department of Nephrology
All India Institute of Medical Sciences Vijaypur
Jammu, J & K

Ashok Kumar Hooda
Senior Consultant, Department of Nephrology
Janakpuri Super Speciality Hospital
New Delhi, India

Ashwani Gupta
Senior Consultant, Department of Nephrology
Sir Ganga Ram Hospital
New Delhi, India

Atul Srivastava
Consultant Nephrologist
Command Hospital (SC)
Pune, Maharashtra, India

Ayan Dey
Consultant Nephrologist
PD Hinduja Hospital
Mumbai, Maharashtra, India

Balasubramaniam Jeyaraj
Senior Consultant Nephrologist & HOD
Kidney Care Centre
Tirunelveli, Tamil Nadu, India

Bhupesh Kumar Saini
Consultant Nephrologist
Command Hospital (CC)
Lucknow, Uttar Pradesh, India

Debasish Mahapatra
Consultant Nephrologist
Command Hospital Air Force
Bengaluru, Karnataka, India

Dharmendra S Bhadauria
Professor, Department of Nephrology
SGPGIMS
Lucknow, Uttar Pradesh, India

Dharshan Rangaswamy
Professor and Head, Department of Nephrology
Kasturba Hospital and Medical College, Manipal
Academy, Udupi, Karnataka, India

Dinesh Khullar
Chairman and HOD, Nephrology
Max Super Speciality Hospital, Saket
New Delhi, India

Dipankar Bhowmik
Professor and Head, Department of Nephrology
All India Institute of Medical Sciences
New Delhi, India

Garima Agarwal
Consultant Nephrologist
Manipal Hospital (Varthur Road)
Bengaluru, Karnataka, India

Gaurav Batta
Consultant Nephrologist
Command Hospital (WC)
Chandigarh, Chandigarh (UT)

Gireesh Reddy G
Assistant Professor, Department of Nephrology
Institute of Nephro Urology
Bengaluru, Karnataka, India

Gurleen Kaur
Nephrologist, Integrative Medicine Specialist
Northeast Georgia Medical Center Gainesville
Georgia, USA

Harbir Singh Kohli
Professor and Head, Department of Nephrology
Postgraduate Institute of Medical Education and Research, Chandigarh, Chandigarh (UT)

Hemant Mehta
Consultant and HOD, Nephrology
Lilavati Hospital and Research Centre
Mumbai, Maharashtra, India

Himanshu Sharma
Associate Professor and HOD, Nephrology
Gandhi Medical College
Bhopal, Madhya Pradesh, India

Indradip Maity
Consultant Nephrologist
Apollo Multispeciality Hospital (Kankurgachi)
Kolkata, West Bengal, India

Indranil Ghosh
Consultant, Department of Nephrology
Army Hospital (R&R)
New Delhi, India

Jai Inder Singh
Consultant Nephrologist
Command Hospital (EC)
Kolkata, West Bengal, India

Jairam A
Professor, Department of Nephrology
St Johns Medical College Hospital
Bengaluru, Karnataka, India

Jithu Kurian
Assistant Professor, Department of Nephrology
Pushpagiri Medical College
Thiruvalla, Kerala, India

Jyothipriya Jyothindrakumar
Consultant Nephrologist
MGM Muthoot Medical Centre
Pathanamthitta, Kerala

Kamal Sud
Clinical Associate Professor & Director, Nephrology
University of Sydney's Nepean Clinical School
Sydney, Australia

Kishore Kumar A
Consultant Nephrologist
PACE Hospitals
Hyderabad, Telangana, India

Kristin George
Consultant Nephrologist
Aster Whitefield Hospital
Bengaluru, Karnataka, India

KS Nayak
Senior Consultant and HOD, Nephrology
Virinchi Hospital
Hyderabad, Telangana, India

KV Baliga
Consultant, Department of Nephrology
ESI Medical College and Hospital
Chennai, Tamil Nadu, India

Manas Ranjan Behera
Associate Professor, Department of Nephrology
Sanjay Gandhi Postgraduate Institute of Medical Sciences, Lucknow, Uttar Pradesh, India

Manas Ranjan Patel
Associate Professor Nephrology
Sanjay Gandhi Post Graduate Institute of Medical Sciences, Lucknow, Uttar Pradesh, India

Manish R Balwani
Consultant, Department of Nephrology
Saraswati Kidney Care Centre
Nagpur, Maharashtra, India

Mohan V Bhojaraja
Associate Professor, Department of Nephrology
Kasturba Hospital and Medical College, Manipal Academy, Udupi, Karnataka, India

Mohd Aslam
Professor and In charge, Nephrology
Jawaharlal Nehru Medical College
Aligarh, Uttar Pradesh, India

Narayan Prasad
Professor and Head, Department of Nephrology
Sanjay Gandhi Postgraduate Institute of Medical Sciences, Lucknow, Uttar Pradesh, India

Narinder Pal Singh
Academic Consultant, Department of Nephrology
Max Super Speciality Hospital, Saket
New Delhi, India

Naveen Mattewada
Consultant Nephrologist
Virinchi Hospital
Hyderabad, Telangana, India

Naveen Medi
Consultant Nephrologist
Virinchi Hospital
Hyderabad, Telangana, India

Nikesh Agrawal
Consultant Nephrologist
INHS Kalyani
Visakhapatnam, Andhra Pradesh, India

Nikhil Bhasin
Consultant Nephrologist
Nanavati Max Super Speciality Hospital
Mumbai, Maharashtra, India

Pavitra Manu Dogra
Professor, Department of Nephrology
Army Hospital (R&R)
New Delhi, India

Prabhat Chauhan
Consultant Nephrologist
INHS Asvini
Mumbai, Maharashtra, India

Pranith Ram M
Consultant Nephrologist
Yashodha Hospital
Hyderabad, Telangana, India

Prem P Varma
Senior Consultant Head, Department of Nephrology
Primus Hospital
New Delhi, India

Priti Meena
Assistant Professor, Department of Nephrology
All India Institute of Medical Sciences
Bhubaneshwar, Odisha, India

Raj Kunwar Yadav
Additional Professor, Department of Nephrology
All India Institute of Medical Sciences
New Delhi, India

Ramanjit Singh Akal
Consultant, Department of Nephrology
7 Air Force Hospital
Kanpur, Uttar Pradesh, India

Ranjith Kumar Nair
Professor Nephrology
Army Hospital (R&R) & O/o DGAFMS
New Delhi, India

Rashmi Yadav
Consultant Nephrologist
MGM Hospital Vashi
Navi Mumbai, Maharashtra, India

Sachin Srivastava
Consultant Nephrologist
Command Hospital (NC)
Udhampur, J&K, India

Sambit Sundaray
Consultant Nephrologist
Command Hospital Air Force
Bengaluru, Karnataka, India

Sanjeev Nair
Consultant Nephrologist
Madras Medical Mission Hospital
Chennai Tamil Nadu, India

Sandeep Mahajan
Professor, Department of Nephrology
All India Institute of Medical Sciences
New Delhi, India

Sanjay Panda
Consultant Nephrologist
Base Hospital Delhi Cantt
New Delhi, India

Sayali Thakare
Associate Professor, Department of Nephrology
GS Medical College and KEM Hospital
Mumbai, Maharashtra, India

Shahbaj Zia Salari
Resident, Department of Nephrology
Jawaharlal Nehru Medical College
Aligarh, Uttar Pradesh, India

Shahbaj Ahmad
Consultant Nephrologist
Himalayan Institute of Medical Sciences
Dehradun, UK

Shaurya Kaul
PhD Scholar, Faculty of Behavioural Sciences
Shree Guru Gobind Singh Tricentenary
University, Gurugram, Haryana, India

Shourya Mohakud
Senior Resident, Department of Nephrology
Sanjay Gandhi Postgraduate Institute of Medical
Sciences, Lucknow, Uttar Pradesh, India

Shyam Bihari Bansal
Director and Head, Department of Nephrology
Medanta—The Medicity Hospital
Gurugram, Haryana, India

Smriti Sinha
Consultant Nephrologist
Marengo Asia Hospital
Faridabad, Haryana, India

Sourabh Sharma
Assistant Professor, Department of Nephrology
VMMC and Safdarjung Hospital
New Delhi, India

Sree Bhusan Raju
Professor and Head, Department of Nephrology
Nizam Institute of Medica Sciences
Hyderabad, Telangana, India

Sudeep Prakash
Consultant Nephrologist
Command Hospital (SC)
Pune, Maharashtra, India

Sukhwinder Singh Sangha
Consultant Nephrologist
Command Hospital (CC)
Lucknow, Uttar Pradesh, India

Subho Banerjee
Associate Professor, Department of Nephrology
Institute of Kidney Diseases and Research Center
Ahmedabad, Gujarat, India

Sumita Bhogal
Consultant Nephrologist
Alchemist Hospital
Panchkula, Haryana, India

Tomala Murari
Consultant Nephrologist
Military Hospital Jalandhar
Jalandhar, Punjab, India

Umesh B Khanna
Senior Consultant Nephrologist and Director
Kidney Associates
Mumbai, Maharashtra, India

Urmila Anandh
Senior Consultant Head, Department of Nephrology
Amrita Hospital
Faridabad, Haryana, India

Vijoy Kumar Jha
Consultant Nephrologist
Base Hospital Delhi Cantt
New Delhi, India

Vinant Bhargava
Consultant, Department of Nephrology
Sir Ganga Ram Hospital
New Delhi, India

Vineet Behera
Consultant Nephrologist
INHS Kalyani
Visakhapatnam, Andhra Pradesh, India

Vishal Singh
Professorand Head, Department of Nephrology
Army Hospital (R&R)
New Delhi, India

Vivek Kute
Professor, Department of Nephrology
Institute of Kidney Diseases and Research Center
Ahmedabad, Gujarat, India

Foreword

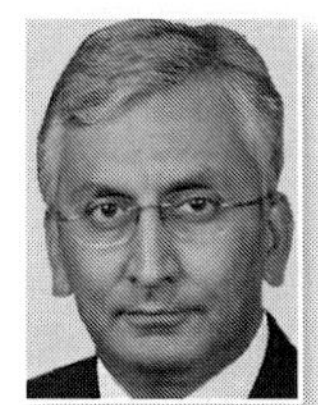

Dialysis medicine is one of the most essential, rapidly evolving, and complex fields of medicine. All healthcare workers involved in dialysis, namely the nephrologists, dialysis physicians, and dialysis nurse or technician must be well versed with all aspects of this advancing field of medicine. In fact, the technicians and the nurses working in dialysis units are the ones whom the patients meet and interact with more frequently, start the dialysis procedure, supervise the entire process, and deal with most complications.

The patient's satisfaction and outcomes of dialysis largely depend on how the healthcare workers manage the dialysis. There is a genuine knowledge gap in the training imparted to the dialysis technicians in terms of good academic knowledge, understanding of pathophysiology of diseases, knowing the engineering and technical aspects of dialysis machines, and in being aware of other linked aspects of nephrology like kidney transplant, or peritoneal dialysis. Therefore, it is imperative to train the technician in various additional aspects of nephrology including physiology, pathology of diseases, basic of therapeutic interventions, infection control, nutrition, to enable him in providing comprehensive medical care.

This book for dialysis technicians is an ideal resource to bridge this gap. The editors and the authors must be congratulated for their efforts in creating this comprehensive book. This laudable effort will be certainly of immense value to our technician and nurse colleagues. The book aims to provide them with the required knowledge in a simplified language which they would be able to understand, with an adequate blend of academic knowledge and practical application, encompassing all the aspects which a technician may come across.

They will be able to enrich themselves with fundamentals of the function of the kidney, the manifestations of kidney failure, and the technical aspects of not only dialysis and water treatment, but also other extracorporeal techniques that are commonly undertaken by the same workforce. They will also learn about other components of kidney replacement therapy including kidney transplantation and peritoneal dialysis. I do hope that the community for whom this resource is intended will find value and provide feedback to the editors and authors that the next editions are even more to their liking.

Vivekanand Jha
MD DM FRCP FAMS
Executive Director, Geroge Institute, India
Past President, International Society of Nephrology
Editor-in-Chief, Indian Journal of Nephrology

Prologue

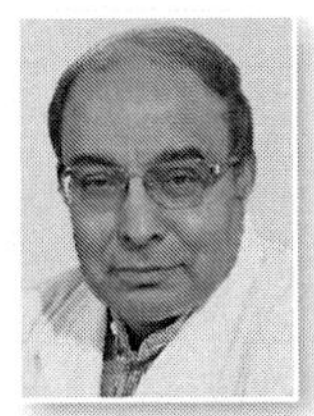

The field of Nephrology and Dialysis has considerably evolved over the years. The erstwhile primitive dialysis machines have made way for the advanced modern and accurate dialysis machines, which are more effective and patient oriented. Dialysis also involves related topics like vascular access creation and care, interventional nephrology, modifications like hemodiafiltration, extracorporeal therapies, creation of ultra-pure RO water, and kidney transplant as a better alternative whenever feasible. It has therefore become imperative for all healthcare workers involved in dialysis, to update their knowledge and stay abreast of the various aspects of dialysis. A patient on maintenance hemodialysis visits dialysis unit 100–150 times a year and thus dialysis staff develops a close emotional and medical association with each dialysis patient and they become friends forever.

Dialysis providers involve dialysis technicians or nurses, and they constitute the key link between the nephrologist and the dialysis patient. They actively interact and provide regular care to the patient, and are involved at most stages of patient interaction. The present-day technician has to perform several vital roles apart from just providing dialysis. He/She has to identify and manage complications, keep the dialysis machines and RO plant functioning well, know the engineering of these equipments to ensure proper maintenance, counsel the patient about dialysis related complications, provide dietary advice, look after and identify problems in vascular access, and timely counsel the patient for kidney transplant. This is only possible by EMPOWERING the dialysis technicians with the sound academic and practical knowledge of all aspects of dialysis and nephrology, such as anatomy, physiology, pathology of diseases, drug information, rationale of interventions, clinical medicine, and nutrition. In the current digital age, quantifying delivered dose of dialysis and auditing the dialysis outcomes on regular basis should become a norm in every good dialysis unit. One can diagnose complications early and manage them effectively. These are likely to be picked up and intervened early.

The Textbook for Dialysis Technicians edited by Dr Narinder Pal Singh and Dr Vineet Behera, with contributions from renowned national and international authors, is an excellent resource for dialysis technicians/nurses. The chapters strike a perfect balance between academic knowledge, practical application, hands-on skills, and put together in a concise, easy to understand chapters. I congratulate the editors and the authors, and hope that this unique endeavor is successful in achieving the mission of imparting knowledge and training to dialysis care providers, to achieve better nephrology care for the patients.

Vijay Kher
DNB DM MNAMS
Chairman
Department of Nephrology
Epitome Kidney Urology Institute
New Delhi, India

Preface

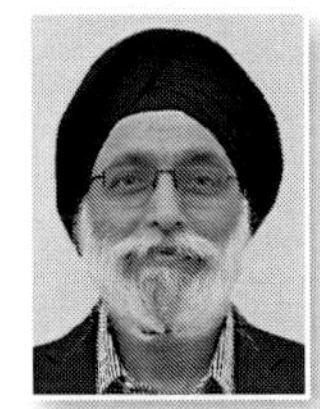

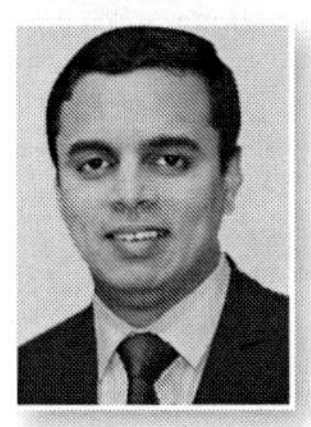

Dialysis has evolved substantially over the years to transform into an entire specialty. It encompasses a large spectrum involving kidney medicine, physiology, pharmacology, general medicine, infectious diseases, surgery, with knowledge of technology, engineering, hygiene sanitation, and various other aspects. A dialysis technician needs to be well-versed with all these aspects to be a successful dialysis provider. Moreover, dialysis entails various attributes of academic knowledge, decision making, clinical aptitude, surgical skills, and social interaction. Therefore, while training dialysis technicians, it is essential to achieve a balance between scholarship, clarity, and practicality. The present-day technician cannot be limited to dialysis only but is frequently exposed to other fields, such as kidney transplantation, peritoneal dialysis, interventional nephrology, nutrition, and others.

The *Textbook for Dialysis Technicians* has been designed keeping all the above aspects in mind. This covers the academic curriculum for dialysis technicians by covering most topics from the syllabus for dialysis training from various universities of the country. The book also emphasizes on bedside and hands-on knowledge by covering the practical aspects of dialysis. The various technical, engineering, or administrative aspects of dialysis are also discussed to provide a holistic knowledge of dialysis. Every effort has been made to provide an overview of additional components of nephrology, to which a dialysis technician is exposed.

The chapters in the book are authored by nationally and internationally acclaimed nephrologists who are the expert in the field. The chapters bring together a blend of academic knowledge, evidence-based medicine pearls of their experience, and key clinical insights, making it a great resource. The chapters have been planned with the requirement of a dialysis technician in mind. However, any further knowledge on a particular topic may be sought by going through the suggested readings at the end of each chapter.

We would like to thank all of our wonderful contributing authors who have spent countless hours in producing high-quality, up-to-date information. On behalf of all the contributors, we sincerely hope that our efforts will contribute to making this book a valuable reference and guide for dialysis technicians. It is through the accomplishment of these objectives, we hope that the dialysis therapy will improve so that the quality of life for all of our patients with kidney disease may improve.

Narinder Pal Singh
Vineet Behera

Acknowledgments

"Guru Brahma Guru Vishnu Guru Devo Maheshwaraha
Guru Saakshat Para Brahma Tasmai Shree Gurave Namaha"

The famous Sanskrit verse means—the Guru (teacher) is the very representative of Supreme God in the Universe (Brahma, Vishnu, and Shiva). He creates and sustains knowledge and destroys the weeds of ignorance. I salute you, the Guru (teacher).

At the outset, with this quote we wish to thank all our teachers of the past, present, and future who have taught us Medicine and Nephrology or anything in life, which has made us capable enough to write this book.

We extend our heartfelt gratitude to all national and international authors who are experts in their field and have taken time off from their busy schedule, to share their knowledge and experience, in their chapters.

We could complete this task only with the constant unwavering support and encouragement of our families and friends. We also thank our colleagues and co-faculty of our departments in supporting us through this educational initiative.

We are also indebted to our publishers—Shri Jitendar P Vij (Group Chairman), Mr Ankit Vij (Managing Director), Mr MS Mani (Group President), Dr Madhu Choudhary (Director—Educational Publishing), Ms Pooja Bhandari [Director-Production (Books and Journals)], Ms Sunita Katla (EA to Group Chairman and Publishing Manager), Ms Samina Khan (EA to Director—Educational Publishing), Dr Upma Tomar (Development Editor), Mr Ajay Kumar Sharma [DGM (Books and Journals)], Ms Seema Dogra (Cover Visualizer), Ms Neha Verma (Graphic Designer—Cover), Mr Rajesh Sharma (Production Coordinator), Mr Vakil Khan (Proofreader), Mr Jagvir Singh Tomar (Typesetter), and Mr Gopal Kirola (Graphic Designer) who involved in the production process.

Contents

Appendices

PLATE 1

Classification of CKD using GFR and ACR Categories

GFR and ACR categories and risk of adverse outcomes			ACR categories (mg/mmol), description and range		
			<3 Normal to mildly increased	3–30 Normal to mildly increased	>30 Severely increased
			A1	A2	A3
GFR categories [mL/min/1.73 m²], description and range	≥90 Normal and high	G1	No CKD in the absence of markers of kidney damage		
	60–89 Mild reduction related to normal range for a young adult	G2			
	45–59 Mild–moderatre reduction	G3a[1]			
	30–44 moderate-severe reduction	G3b			
	15–29 Severe reduction	G4			
	<15 Kidney failure	G5			

Increasing risk (down the GFR categories)

Increasing risk (across the ACR categories)

PLATE 2

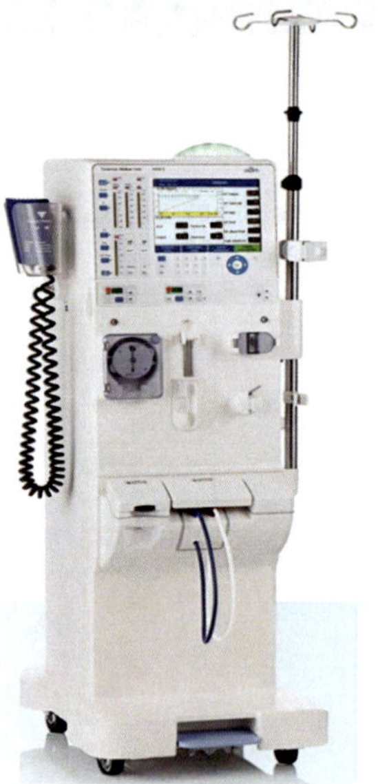

Hemodialysis Machine
(4008 S Classix, Fresenius Medical care)

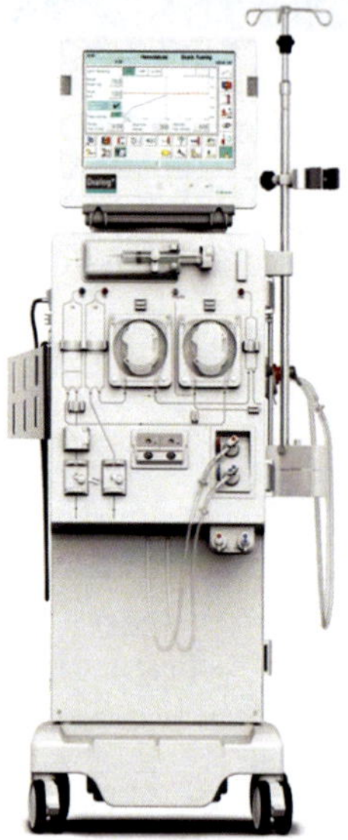

Hemodiafiltration Machine
(B Braun Dialog +)

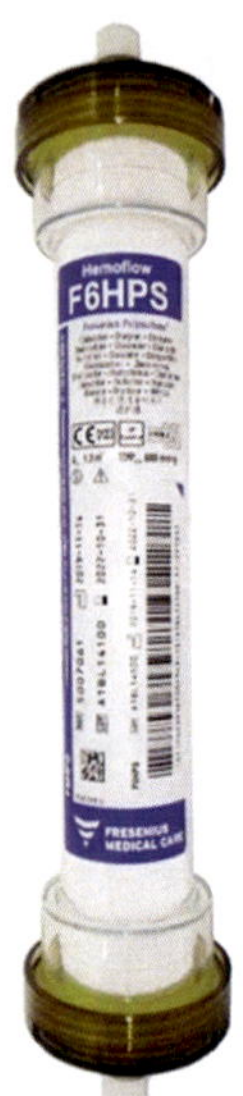

Hemodialyzer

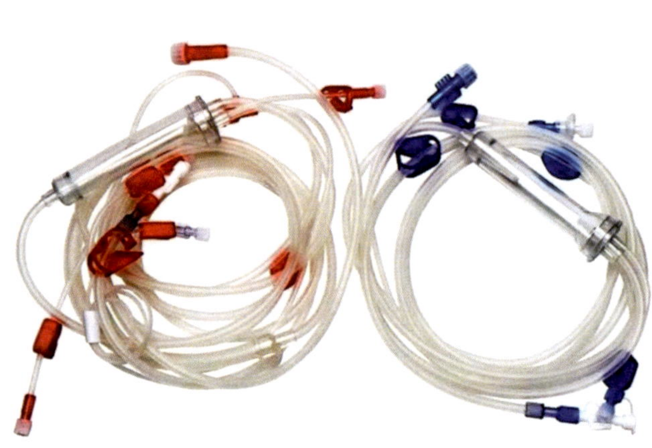

Blood tubings

PLATE 3

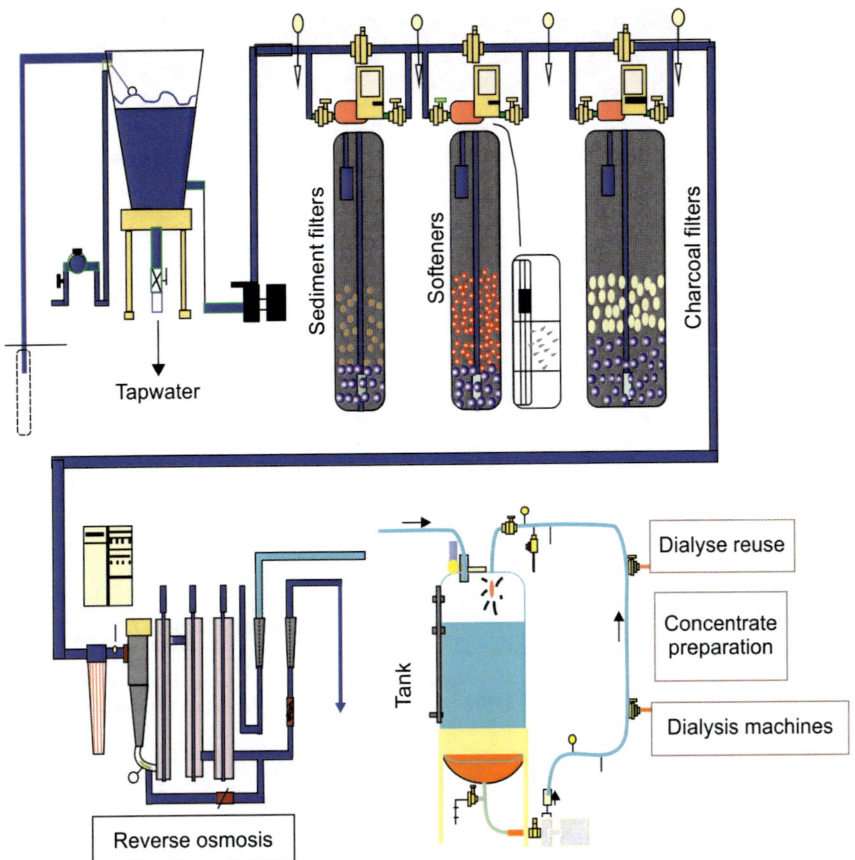

Schematic diagram—RO water plant for dialysis

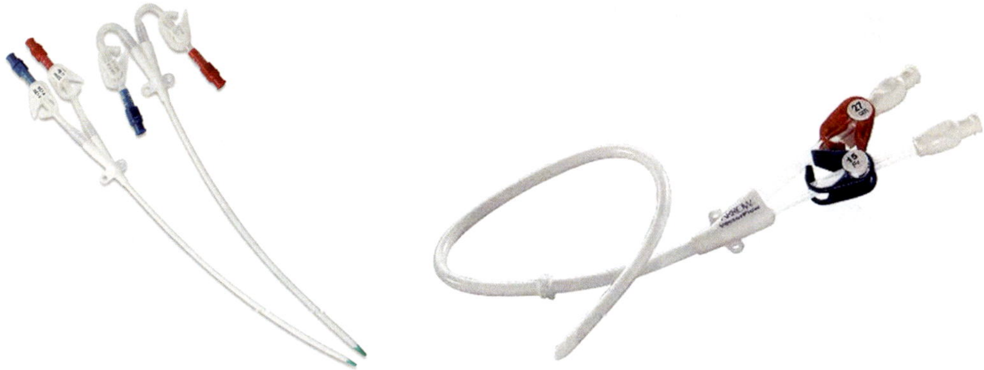

Temporary dialysis catheters (Straight and coiled)

Tunneled cuffed dialysis catheters

PLATE 4

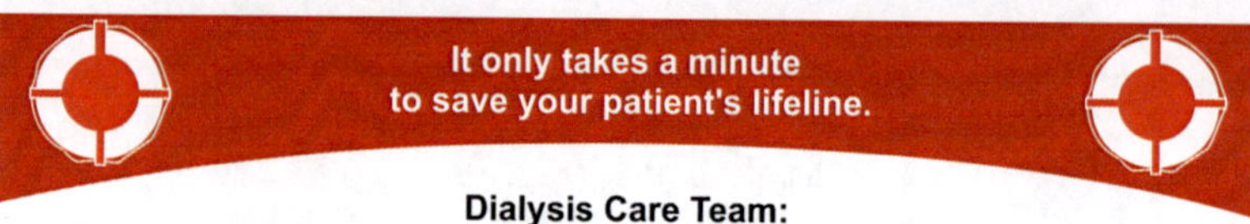

It only takes a minute
to save your patient's lifeline.
Dialysis Care Team:
• Perform access check at each treatment or when patient reports a change.
• Reinforce importance of daily access checks to patient.
• Listen to the patient.
Look
Listen
Feel
Arm elevation test (AVF only)
Augmentation test (Optional)

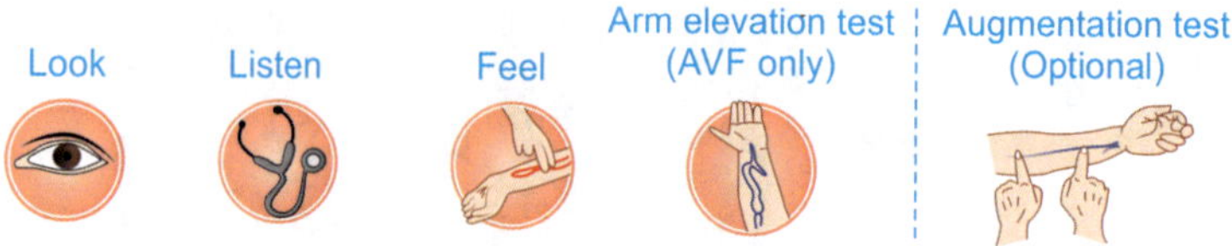

2 min AV fistula bedside examination

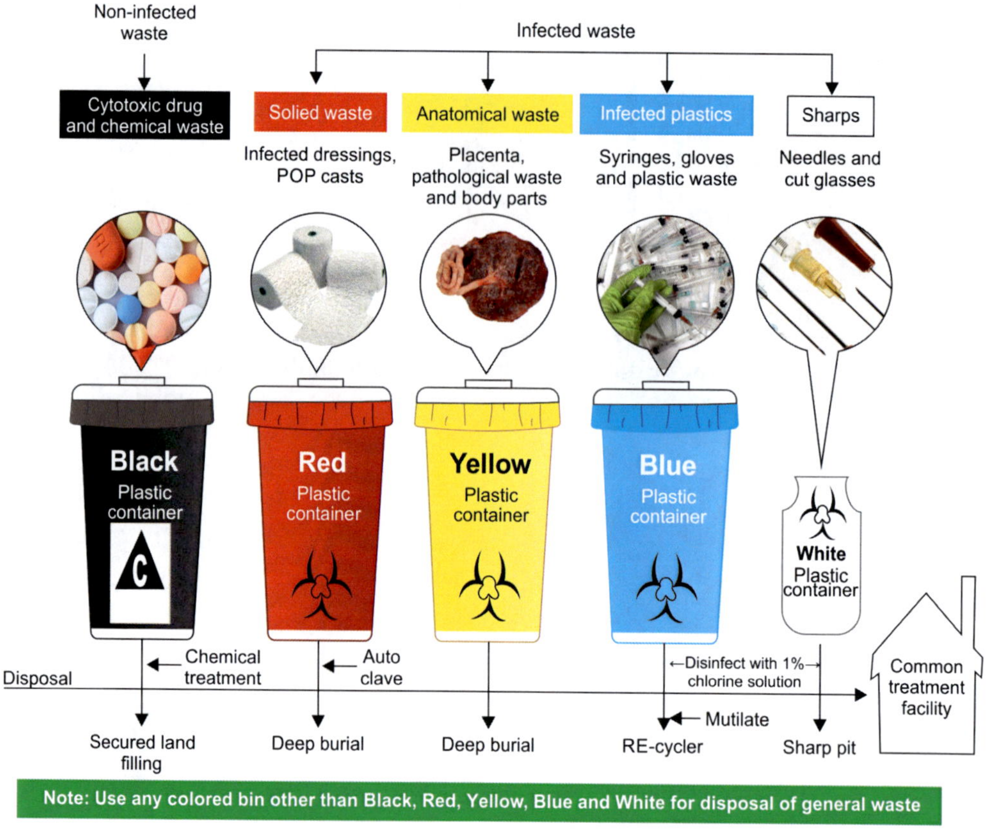

Non-infected waste
Infected waste
Cytotoxic drug and chemical waste
Solied waste
Anatomical waste
Infected plastics
Sharps
Infected dressings, POP casts
Placenta, pathological waste and body parts
Syringes, gloves and plastic waste
Needles and cut glasses
Black
Plastic container
C
Red
Plastic container
Yellow
Plastic container
Blue
Plastic container
White
Plastic container
Disposal
Chemical treatment
Auto clave
Disinfect with 1% chlorine solution
Mutilate
Common treatment facility
Secured land filling
Deep burial
Deep burial
RE-cycler
Sharp pit
Note: Use any colored bin other than Black, Red, Yellow, Blue and White for disposal of general waste

Management of solid biomedical wastes

PLATE 5

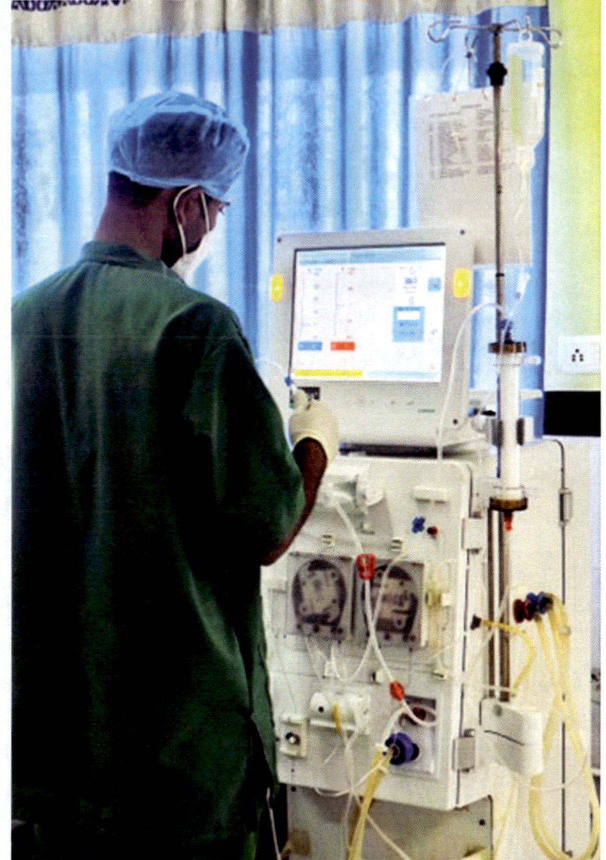

Fig. 4: Priming being undertaken on a B Braun Dialog + machine with dialyser and tubing already connected. Note that dialyser couplings and concentrate line couplings are attached with the machine at this point.

PLATE 6

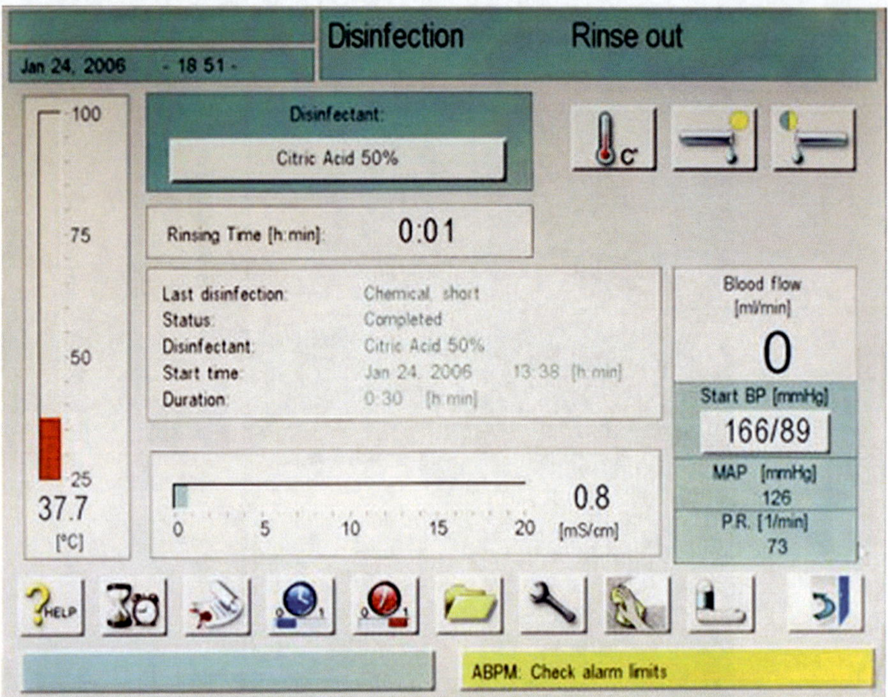

Fig. 1: Disinfection options in a B Braun Dialog + HD machine. Note options of thermal, full and short chemical disinfections. If none of the options are selected, then the machine remains in 'Rinse Mode' and during this internal circuits are rinsed or washed with ultrapure water.

PLATE 7

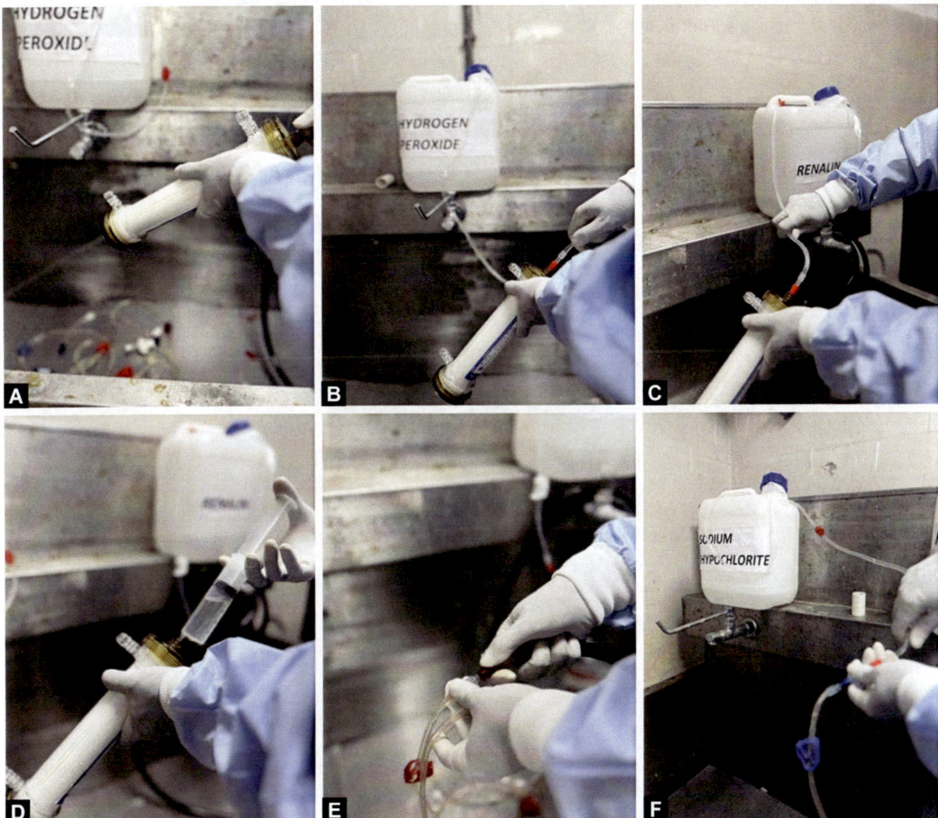

Figs. 1A to F: (A) Manual washing: Flushing of dialyser with RO water; (B) Filling of hydrogen peroxide in dialyser; (C) Measuring total cell volume using 50 mL syringe; (D) Filling of renalin; (E) AV tubing flushing with RO water; (F) Filling of sodium hypochlorite solution in AV tubing.

PLATE 8

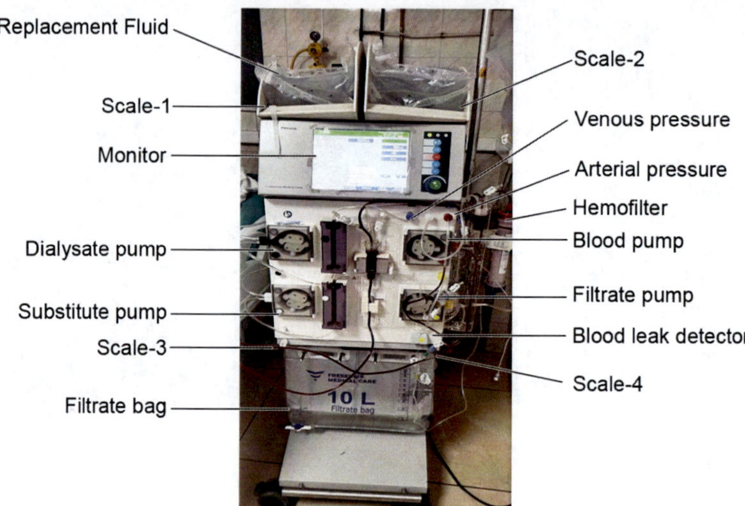

Fig. 2: Machine for continuous renal replacement therapy.

Anatomy and Physiology of Kidneys

1
CHAPTER

Sourya Sourabh Mohakuda, Vineet Behera, Ashwani Gupta

ANATOMY OF KIDNEYS

Kidneys are a pair of bean shaped organ enveloped by their respective capsule in the posterior aspect of lumbar region of abdomen. They together weigh around 300 g and are 9–11 cm in length, equivalent to roughly length of three lumbar vertebra. The right kidney is situated slightly lower than the left kidney. Each kidney is further divided into outer cortex and inner medulla. Kidney is a collection of nephrons and each nephron is further divided into glomerulus, tubules and collecting duct **(Fig. 1)**. The kidneys are connected to the bladder by ureters on either side.

Vascular Supply and Control of Blood Flow

Kidneys are supplied by a pair of renal arteries and drained by a pair of renal veins, one on either side. The renal artery further subdivides into interlobar, interlobular and arcuate arteries within the kidney **(Fig. 2)**. The smallest branch of the artery forms the afferent vessels of the glomerulus which is the filtration unit of the kidney. The glomerulus receives 20% of cardiac output in a day, and receives 600 mL/min blood flow. Of this, only 20%, i.e., 120 mL/min is filtered out of glomerulus.

The difference in pressure between the afferent and efferent arteriole, i.e., 40 mm Hg is responsible for the filtration across the glomerulus. The constriction of afferent arterioles leads to decrease in glomerular filtration rate (GFR) by decreasing the blood flow to glomerulus.

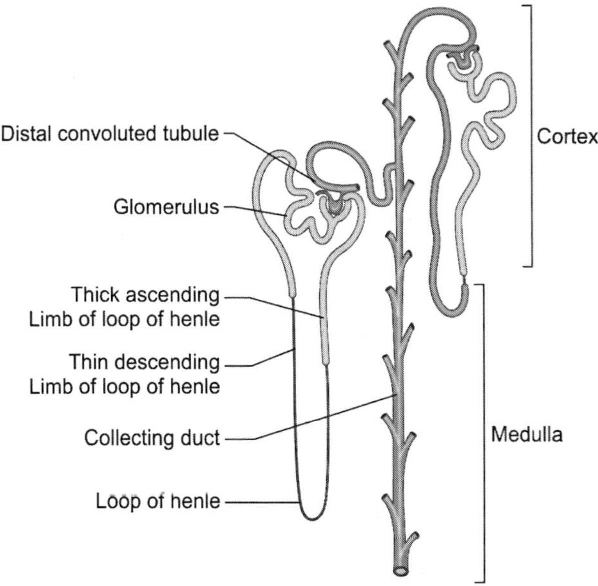

Fig. 1: Anatomy of nephron.

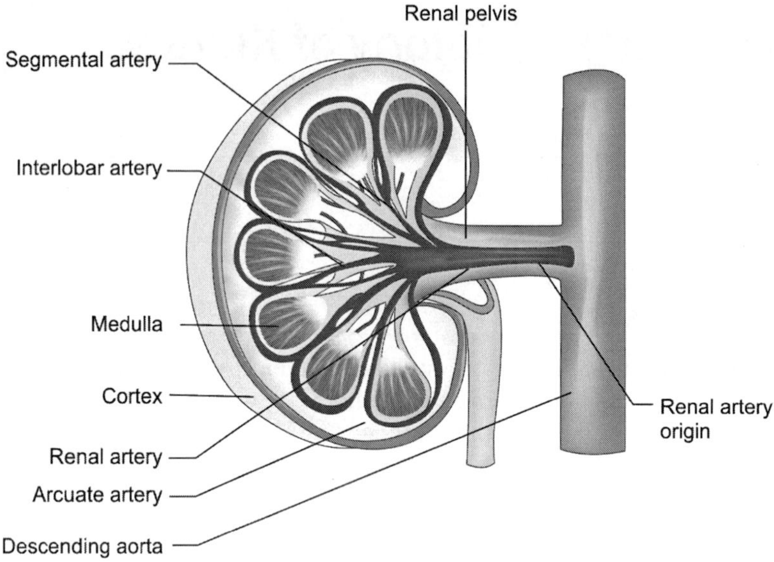

Fig. 2: Arterial supply of kidneys.

Similarly, the relaxation of efferent arteriole leads to decreased GFR by decreased pressure gradient. The afferent and efferent arteriolar diameter is controlled by myogenic reflex and hormones.

Myogenic reflex is the control of blood vessels as per proportional blood flow. If there is increase in blood flow across glomerulus, the reflex system activates to increase the vessel diameter leading to lower pressure and vice versa if there is decreased blood flow.

Hormone primarily responsible for GFR control is angiotensin-II (AT-II) which is responsible for efferent arteriolar constriction. The lesser the efferent arteriolar diameter, more is the GFR. The action of angiotensin II is antagonized by prostaglandins. Other hormones like arginine vasopressin along with AT-II decrease glomerular permeability while prostacycline and atrial natriuretic factor increase the glomerular permeability.

The number of nephrons in kidney also play a role in determining GFR. As age progresses, GFR declines at a rate of 1 mL/min beyond 40 years of age.

PHYSIOLOGY OF KIDNEY

Formation of Urine

After the blood is filtered across the glomerulus, it reaches the tubular part of the nephron. The first part encountered by the filtered fluid is proximal convoluted tubule (PCT). In the PCT, majority of glucose, amino acids and bicarbonate is reabsorbed. Water is also absorbed proportionately to sodium reabsorption leading to iso osmolarity of the resultant fluid. The reabsorption of chloride is less that of bicarbonate leading to a hyperchloremic acidic filtrate recaching the thin part of descending limb of loop of Henle.

The loop of Henle is richly vascular with supply from surrounding vasa recta. It contributes to the maximum water balance of kidneys. The descending limb functions by reabsorption of water along with sodium, potassium and urea. The ascending limb being impermeable to water and permeable to solutes is responsible for creation of hypotonic urine. Further there is exchange of electrolytes from descending limb of vasa recta to the tubules leading which is also called as counter current exchange.

The hypotonic urine reaches the distal convoluted tubule (DCT) followed by collecting duct. In the absence of anti diuretic hormone (ADH) there will be passage of hypotonic urine. Aldosterone and ADH are responsible for the salt and preferential water reabsorption across the DCT and collecting duct making the final urine concentrated.

Role of Renin, Prostaglandins and Kinins

There are specialized cells in the afferent arteriole of the glomerulus known as juxtaglomerular cells which is responsible for the release of renin. Renin acts by activating angiotensin hormone which in turn is responsible for the secretion of aldosterone. Aldosterone is responsible for the sodium and water reabsorption in the kidneys. The sensing of requirements of renin release is by organization of cells acting together which is called the juxtaglomerular apparatus. Juxtaglomerular apparatus consists of the juxtaglomerular cells, specialized sodium concentration sensing cells in the distal tubule (macula densa cells), the efferent arteriole and some part of the interstitium **(Fig. 3)**. When required, juxtaglomerular apparatus is responsible for secreting hormones to regulate the constriction of vessels, control of thirst and release of anti diuretic hormone.

Prostaglandins, leukotrienes and thromboxanes are metabolites of arachidonic acid and control GFR directly by affecting vascular tension and indirectly by interacting with hormones which affect GFR.

Kinins such as bradykinin is released from the distal nephron and is associated with vasodilatory action and stimulating renin release which affects GFR.

Erythropoietin

It is a 45,000 dalton sized glycoprotein which gets activated in the glomerular region of kidney and is responsible for production, maturation and differentiation of red cells in the bone marrow. The primary stimulus for the release of erythropoietin is low oxygen levels in the renal tissue.

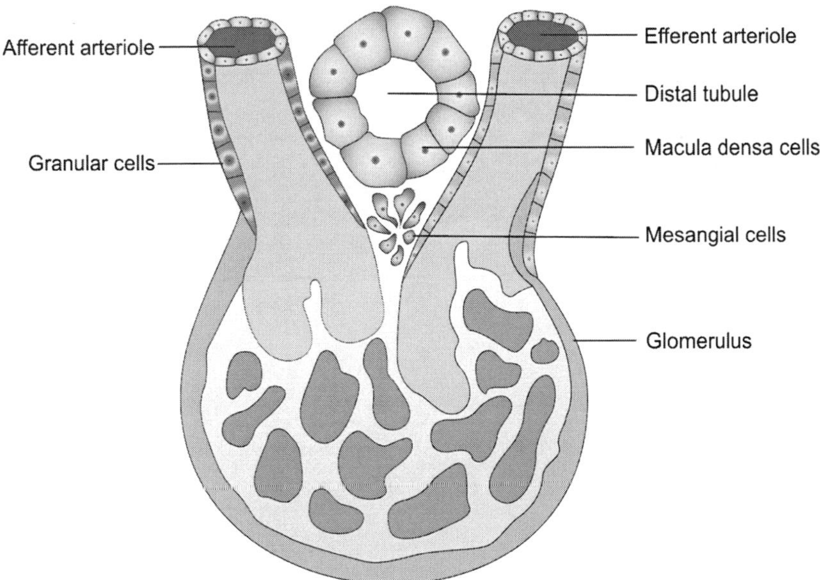

Fig. 3: Anatomy of juxtaglomerular apparatus.

Apart from the above hormones, kidneys also produce an active form of vitamin D, i.e., 1,25 dihydroxy cholecalciferol, which is responsible for absorption of calcium and phosphorus. The production and release of this hormone is predominantly under the control of parathyroid hormone (PTH).

SUGGESTED READING

1. Holechek MJ. Glomerular filtration: An overview. Nephrol Nurs J J Am Nephrol Nurses Assoc. 2003;30(3):285-90; quiz 291-2.
2. Ogobuiro I, Tuma F. Physiology, Renal. In: StatPearls [Internet]. Treasure Island (FL): StatPearls Publishing; 2023.
3. Renal system 1: The anatomy and physiology of the kidneys. Nursing Times [Internet]. [cited 2023 Nov 6].
4. Sahay M, Kalra S, Bandgar T. Renal endocrinology: The new frontier. Indian J Endocrinol Metab. 2012;16(2):154-5.

Common Diseases of Kidney

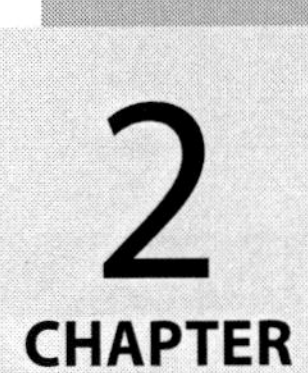

Prabhat Chauhan, A Jairam, Ashok Kumar Hooda

INTRODUCTION

Kidney diseases are quite common and leads to lot of morbidity and mortality. Based on the presentation kidney diseases can be divided into:

- Acute kidney injury
- Chronic kidney disease
- Nephrotic syndrome
- Nephritic syndrome
- Renal stone disease
- Urinary tract obstruction
- Urinary tract infections
- Renal tubule defects
- Hypertension
- Asymptomatic urinary abnormalities.

The symptoms related to kidney **(Fig. 1)** are sometimes correctable leading to cure of hypertension. Primary hypertension is controlled using blood pressure lowering drugs, salt restriction and lifestyle changes.

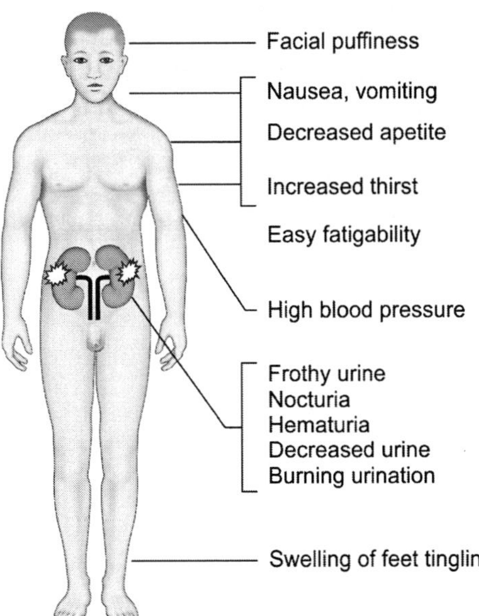

Fig. 1: Common symptoms of kidney disease.

Table 1: Common glomerular disorders.

Primary glomerular disorders	*Secondary glomerular disorders*
Minimal change disease (MCD)	ANCA vasculitis (pauci-immune glomerulonephritis)
Membranous glomerulonephritis (MGN)	Lupus nephritis
Focal segmental glomerulosclerosis (FSGS)	Anti glomerular basement membrane disease
Membrano proliferative glomerulonephritis (MPGN)	IgA vasculitis
IgA nephropathy (IgAN)	

COMMON DISEASES OF KIDNEY

Glomerular Diseases

Disease affecting the glomeruli are usually autoimmune in nature. These can present acutely or can have a very slow smoldering course. If diagnosed early these are potentially treatable. The common symptoms may include frothy urine, dark colored urine and swelling of feet. Glomerular diseases are implicated in up to 8–9% cases of CKD. The common glomerular diseases are given in **Table 1**.

Glomerular diseases can present as nephrotic or nephritic syndrome, while nephrotic syndrome presents with swelling of feet, frothy urine and decreased urine output, nephritic syndrome predominantly presents with dark colored urine, swelling and raised blood pressure. Differentiating between nephrotic and nephritic syndrome **(Table 2)** helps in diagnosis as well as management.

Cystic Disorders or Polycystic Kidneys (Fig. 2)

Cysts are fluid filled cavities in the kidneys. They can be due to a variety of causes. Polycystic kidney diseases (PKD) are a group of genetic diseases that cause cysts to grow in kidneys, liver, pancreas, and spleen. The common genes associated are the PKD1 and PKD 2. The continuous growth of these cysts leads to damage to the normal kidney and ultimately to kidney failure. Brain can also be affected with abnormal dilatation of arteries (aneurysms) which can rupture. Cystic kidney diseases are implicated in up to 3–4% of CKD.

Table 2: Differences between nephrotic and nephritic syndrome.

Typical features	*Nephrotic syndrome*	*Nephritic syndrome*
Onset	Slow	Fast
Edema	++++	++
Blood pressure	Normal	Raised
Proteinuria	++++	++
Hematuria	Unlikely	+++
Serum albumin	Low	Normal to slightly reduced
Common conditions	MCD, FSGS, MGN	IgAN, MPGN, lupus nephritis

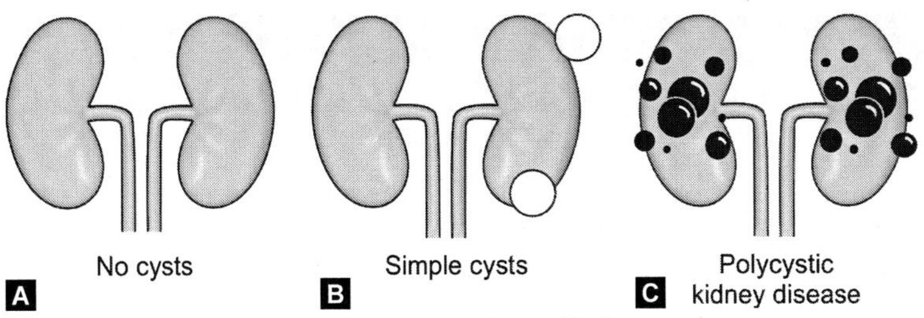

Fig. 2: Cystic disorders of kidney.

Renal Stone Disease

Kidney stones are very common and may be seen in up to 1% of population. Kidney stones are of four main types:

1. Calcium stones
2. Uric acid stones
3. Struvite stones
4. Cysteine stones

Kidney stones can present in variety of ways which include:

- Asymptomatic
- Colicky pain
- Blood in urine
- Kidney infection
- Kidney dysfunction—if bilateral stones.

Imaging tests like X-ray, USG and CT are used to detect the stones. Based on the type, size and number of stones the stones can be treated with lithotripsy, or surgical stone removal.

Urinary Tract Obstruction

Obstruction of urinary tract can be caused by congenital or acquired causes. The common causes of urinary tract obstruction (UTO) include stones, tumors, stricture and bladder dysfunction. Sometimes urinary tract obstruction can be due to congenital causes. UTO can be asymptomatic or may present with pain, decreased urine output, recurrent infections or sometimes even with advanced kidney failure. USG is the most common investigation to diagnose urinary tract obstruction.

Acute Kidney Injury

Acute kidney injury (AKI) is characterized by rapid loss of kidney function. Infections, toxins, dehydration, immunological diseases and obstruction are common causes of AKI.

AKI is further classified into:

1. Prerenal
2. Intrarenal, or
3. Postrenal, based on what part of the excretory system is affected.

- **Prerenal AKI** is caused due to reduced or absent blood flow to the kidneys. This can be because of fluid loss (dehydration, bleeding), heart disease (myocardial infarction leading to low blood pressure) or even due to acute blockade of the arteries supplying the kidneys restoring the blood flow to the kidneys usually leads to rapid improvement of prerenal AKI.

Table 3: Stages of acute kidney injury.	
Stage	**Criteria**
1.	• Increase in creatinine by more than 0.3 mg/dL over 48 hours • Or increase to ≥1.5–1.9 times the reference range
2.	Increase to ≥2–2.9 times the reference range
3.	• Increase to ≥3.0 times the reference range Or • Absolute value more than 4 mg/dL Or • Need for dialysis

- **Intrarenal AKI** is caused by any infection, toxin or immunological diseases. Treatment of the underlying cause (like antibiotics for infections) and supportive therapy to correct any fluid and electrolyte imbalance is the preferred strategy.
- **Postrenal AKI** occurs due to blockage to the urinary drainage form the kidneys. This leads to backpressure on the kidneys leading to damage to the kidneys. The main cause of this blockage are stones, tumors, bladder problems and enlarged prostate gland. If not recognized and treated early this can lead to permanent damage to kidneys (chronic kidney disease).

AKI is associated with a lot of morbidity and mortality. If proper treatment is not given at an early-stage, AKI can progress to chronic kidney disease (CKD). However early aggressive treatment directed to the underlying cause and supportive treatment can help in achieving back the normal kidney function. Any patient suffering from AKI always remains at risk of future AKI. Based on the severity AKI is divided into 3 stages as shown in **Table 3**.

CHRONIC KIDNEY DISEASE

Chronic kidney disease is characterized by permanent damage to the kidneys. It is usually due to a slow, relentless loss of kidney function because of loss of nephrons. Kidneys have a lot of reserve and even loss of more than half of nephrons may not adversely affect an individual. Also, the early symptoms of CKD are very nonspecific and may not occur till a substantial damage has already occurred. The reported prevalence of CKD ranges from 1–13%. Hence CKD is often missed and people come to medical attention with advanced kidney failure. It is therefore recommended to screen for CKD specially in high-risk groups. Screening may pick up the disease at an early stage where treatment to slow the progression can be given.

Treatment of CKD includes the treatment of the underlying cause (like control of diabetes) and kidney supportive medicines (like sodium bicarbonate for acidosis) . It is also important to teach the patient regarding avoiding nephrotoxic drugs like painkillers, over counter medications and alternative medications. Based on the severity CKD (based on estimated GFR) can be divided into five stages as shown in **Table 4**. Once patient reaches CKD stage

Table 4: Stages of chronic kidney disease.	
Stage	**Estimated GFR (eGFR) mL/min/1.73 m^2**
1.	≥90
2.	60–89
3.	30–59
4.	15–29
5.	<15

Table 5: Risk factors for CKD.

Sl. No.	*Clinical factors*
1.	Diabetes
2.	Hypertension
3.	Autoimmune disease including glomerulonephritis
4.	Cystic kidney diseases
5.	Systemic infections
6.	Urinary tract infections
7.	Urinary tract obstruction
8.	Neoplasia
9.	Family history of CKD
10.	Exposure to certain drugs

five and starts developing complications they need kidney replacement therapy in form of hemodialysis or peritoneal dialysis. Renal transplant is the best form of treatment for end stage kidney disease.

Common Causes of CKD

CKD has a number of causes or risk-factors **(Table 5)**. As per US data diabetes, high blood pressure, or glomerular diseases caused more than ¾ of CKD in patients who started dialysis in 2003.

CKD of Unknown Etiology (CKDu)

Certain rural populations in world have very high prevalence of CKD for which the exact cause is not known. CKDu is thought be multifactorial and linked to several environmental toxins. In India examples include Uddanam region in Andhra Pradesh and Tondaimandalam in Tamil Nadu.

SUGGESTED READING

1. Inker LA, Astor BC, Fox CH, Isakova T, Lash JP, Peralta CA, Kurella TM, Feldman HI. KDOQI US commentary on the 2012 KDIGO clinical practice guideline for the evaluation and management of CKD. Am J Kidney Dis. 2014;63(5).
2. Jameson J, Fauci AS, Kasper DL, Hauser SL, Longo DL, Loscalzo J. Harrison's Principles of Internal Medicine, 20th edition. McGraw-Hill Education; 2018.

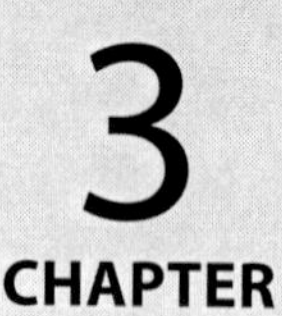

Acute Kidney Injury

3
CHAPTER

Sukhwinder Singh Sangha, Smriti Sinha, Garima Aggarwal

INTRODUCTION

Acute kidney injury (AKI) is defined as an sudden (within 48 hours) fall in kidney function seen as rise in serum creatinine by ≥0.3 mg/dL or reduced urine output of <0.5 mL/kg/h for more than 6 hours.

Acute kidney injury network (AKIN) group categorizes as per the severity of AKI **(Table 1)**. This staging system was previously known as risk, injury, failure, loss, end-stage renal disease (RIFLE).

Table 1: Shows AKIN criteria for AKI.

Stage	*Serum creatinine*	*Urine output*
1.	1.5–1.9 times baseline or ≥0.3 mg/dL increase	<0.5 mL/kg/hr for 6–12 hr
2.	2–2.9 times baseline	<0.5 mL/kg/h for ≥12 hr
3.	3 times baseline OR Increase to ≥4 mg/dL OR Initiation of dialysis	<0.3 mL/kg/hr for ≥24 hr OR Anuria for ≥12 hr

CAUSES AKI

- AKI is divided into prerenal, postrenal, and intrinsic (with in kidney) renal injury as shown in **Table 2**.
- Prerenal AKI refers to problems with renal blood flow, either from decreased intravascular volume, decreased blood pressure, or decrease in effective circulating volume.
- Postrenal AKI is caused by obstruction to urine flow and accounts for ~5–15% of all cases of AKI.
- Intrinsic renal injury can be from glomerular, vascular, interstitial, or tubular compartment of kidney. Acute kidney injury is a common disease of the sick hospitalized patients.
- Sometimes AKI causes no signs or symptoms and is detected as abnormal laboratory tests. Acute kidney injury can be severe and requires intensive treatment. However, acute kidney failure may be reversible if underlying cause can be rectified.

Table 2: Shows the common causes of AKI.

Prerenal causes (reduced blood flow to kidneys)
Blood or fluid loss, e.g., hemorrhage gastroenteritis
Hypotension
Heart failure
Liver failure
Infection related inflammation, cytokine storm, capillary leak syndrome, e.g., dengue
Pain killer like brufen, naproxen, and diclofenac

Contd...

Contd...

Severe burn
Severe dehydration
Intrinsic causes (with in kidneys)
Sepsis related acute kidney injury
Cholesterol emboli that block blood flow in the kidneys following catheterization procedure of major abdominal vessels like coronary angiography
Primary glomerulonephritis (inflammation of the glomeruli)-immune injury to glomeruli, e.g., membranous glomerulonephritis, IgA nephropathy
Infection, such as malaria, leptospira, Hep B, HCV and HIV
Lupus nephritis, an immune disorder causing secondary glomerulonephritis
Medications, chemotherapy drugs, antibiotics and contrast used during imaging tests
Toxins, such as heavy metals and cocaine
Muscle tissue breakdown (rhabdomyolysis) leads to kidney damage by deposition of myoglobin in tubules following severe physical exertion
Breakdown of tumor cells (tumor lysis syndrome) leads to deposition of uric acid and damage to tubules
Clotting of blood in the veins and arteries of the kidneys
Hemolytic uremic syndrome (HUS), a uncommon condition that results from premature destruction of red blood cells and damage to tubules
Postrenal causes (obstruction of urinary tract)
Enlarged prostate
Kidney and urinary tract stones
Blood clots in the urinary tract
Cervical cancer, prostate cancer, and colon cancer
Bladder cancer
Neurogenic (dysfunctional) bladder like diabetic neuropathy, spinal injury

Risk Factors

Acute kidney injury more commonly occurs with another medical condition in sick admitted patients:

- Advanced age
- Diabetes
- High blood pressure
- Heart failure
- Kidney diseases
- Liver diseases
- Certain cancers and their treatments.

Drug induced AKI: Number of drugs like Aminoglycosides (Amikacin), Vancomycin, Amphotericin B, Chemotherapy (Cisplatin), NSIADS (brufen, diclofenac and naproxen) and diuretics have been implicated by either direct injury to tubules or causing vasoconstriction. This form of AKI is more common in elderly, sick and dehydrated patients with other comorbidities.

Contrast induced nephropathy: Iodine-based contrast used in radiology imaging and interventions like coronary angiography is also important cause of AKI. Rise in serum creatinine is seen after 3 days of contrast administration. Contrast induced injury can be minimized by adequate hydration and stopping other nephrotoxic drugs before the procedure.

DIAGNOSIS AKI

Examination of urine: Urinalysis and microscopic examination of the urine sediment is most important test in the evaluation of AKI.

The urinalysis is bland (does not reveal protein, blood, cells, or casts) in prerenal azotemia and in uncomplicated postrenal failure. The urinalysis and sediment may help to not only separate renal causes from pre and postrenal etiologies but also to differentiate between a tubular, glomerular, or interstitial disease conditions. Like presence of RBC cast and dysmorphic RBC are strongly suggestive of glomerular diseases.

If the urine dipstick tests strongly positive for blood but no red blood cells are seen on microscopy, myoglobin or hemoglobin in urine should be suspected, suggesting rhabdomyolysis or severe intravascular hemolysis leading to AKI.

Blood chemistry will reveal elevated urea and creatinine. Elevated plasma blood urea nitrogen out of proportion to serum creatinine (>20:1) should prompt an investigation towards pre renal causes.

Renal ultrasonography is required to diagnose urinary obstruction and planning renal biopsy Renal biopsy is usually done to diagnose intrinsic renal diseases particularly diseases of glomeruli and interstitial compartment.

Complications

Potential complications of acute kidney failure may include:

- Fluid overload in lungs, which can cause shortness of breath.
- **Chest pain:** Inflammation of the lining that covers your heart (pericardium)
- **Muscle weakness:** Body's fluids and electrolytes imbalance can result in muscle weakness.
- **Permanent kidney damage:** Occasionally, acute kidney failure causes permanent loss of kidney function, or end-stage renal disease.
- Acute kidney failure can lead to loss of kidney function and death.

TREATMENT AKI

- Management of AKI depends on the underlying cause.
- Avoidance of additional nephrotoxic agents and further hypotension can hasten renal recovery. Adequate hydration and volume resuscitation will reverse prerenal causes. In liver disease administration of albumin will be helpful for recovery of renal functions.
- **Acid-base, fluid and electrolyte disturbances:** Hyperkalemia and metabolic acidosis are common indications to initiate dialysis. Rhabdomyolysis and tumor lysis syndrome require good hydration initially. Immune-mediated diseases like glomerulonephritis may require immunosuppressant drugs like steroids.
- Any obstruction of urinary tract should be relieved by procedures like placing foley's catheter, suprapubic catheterization of bladder, placement of stents in ureters and percutaneous drain into kidneys.
- **Nutritional support:** Nutrition is one of the important aspect of supportive care. AKI is a stressful, catabolic state, and adequate nutrition is essential with oral or parenteral (intravenous) support and should be initiated in a timely manner. Unlike CKD, where protein restriction is recommended, protein requirements in AKI vary from 1.0 g/kg (prior to dialysis initiation) to 2.5 g/kg in continuous therapy (CRRT).

Dose Adjustment of Medications

Adjusting doses of medications to the GFR is essential in preventing further renal injury as well as avoiding systemic toxicity. Doses and timing is further adjusted when the patient is on HD or CRRT.

Prevention

Acute kidney failure is often difficult to predict or prevent.

- Avoid pain medications
- Proper medical treatment of kidney and other chronic conditions like T2DM, HTN, heart failure and chronic liver disease
- Adopt a healthy lifestyle, regular exercises, maintain ideal body weight and avoid smoking.

SUGGESTED READING

1. Bellomo R, Ronco C, Kellum JA, Mehta RL, Palevsky P. Acute renal failure—definition, outcome measures, animal models, fluid therapy and information technology needs: The Second International Consensus Conference of the Acute Dialysis Quality Initiative (ADQI) Group. Crit Care. 2004;8:R204-12.
2. KDIGO. Clinical Practice Guideline for Acute Kidney Injury. Kidney Int Suppl 2012;2:(8).
3. Mehta RL, Kellum JA, Shah SV, Molitoris BA, Ronco C, Warnock DG, et al. Acute Kidney Injury Network: Report of an initiative to improve outcomes in acute kidney injury. Crit Care. 2007;11:R31.

4
CHAPTER

Chronic Kidney Disease

Sukhwinder Singh Sangha, M Pranith Ram, Sree Bhusan Raju

INTRODUCTION

Kidneys are very important organs of body which filter nitrogen waste product and excess fluids from body, maintain electrolyte, acid base balance and perform various metabolic and endocrine functions in body. Chronic kidney disease (CKD) result from gradual loss of kidney function. CKD is defined as abnormalities of kidney structure or function, present for 3 months, with implications for health. Functional abnormalities include those of blood (raised serum creatinine), urine (protein loss in urine) and structural abnormalities as seen on imaging (small, dysplastic or polycystic kidneys on ultrasonography). CKD is classified into stages **(Fig. 1)** based on mainly estimated glomerular filtration rate (eGFR).

Lately proteinuria component is also added. GFR is calculated by creatinine-based formulas. These formula include Cockroft Gault, Modified Diet in Renal Disease (MDRD) formula, CKD EPI equation. Online calculator are available which calculate GFR from serum creatinine, weight, age, gender and ethnicity. Creatinine is derived from muscle mass and there are so many factors which control serum creatinine other than GFR. So estimating renal functions from creatinine may be misleading in different conditions like extreme of age, weight, muscle mass and pregnancy. In the early stages of chronic kidney disease (stage 1–3) there may be no symptoms. Advanced chronic kidney disease (stage 4–5) can cause dangerous levels of fluid, electrolytes and waste to build up in the body. Most of complication occur at this stage. Patient is also advised for creation of vascular access (arteriovenous fistula).

CLINICAL FEATURES OF CHRONIC KIDNEY DISEASE

Signs and symptoms of chronic kidney disease develop as renal failure progresses and depends upon stage of CKD, as shown in **Figure 2**. These include:

- Nausea, vomiting and loss of appetite
- Fatigue and weakness
- Sleep problems
- Nocturia or oliguria
- Mental slowness and forgetfulness

Stage 1	Stage 2	Stage 3A	Stage 3B	Stage 4	Stage 5
GFR≥90	89≥GFR≥60	59≥GFR≥40	44≥GFR≥30	29≥GFR≥15	GFR<15
Normal or high function	Mildly decreased function	Mild to moderately decreased function		Severely decreased function	Kidney failure

Fig. 1: Stages of chronic kidney disease.

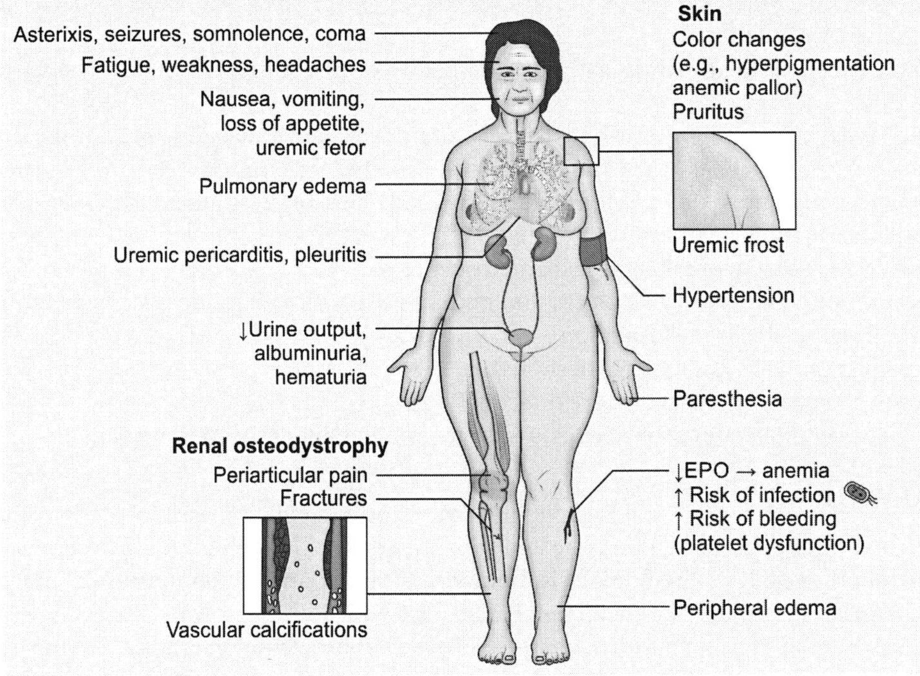

Fig. 2: Shows the symptoms and signs of chronic kidney disease.

(*Source:* Adapted from Davidosn's Principles of Internal Medicine)

- Muscle cramps
- Swelling of feet and ankles
- Dry and itchy skin
- New onset or worsening of hypertension
- Shortness of breath
- Chest pain
- Sexual dysfunction

CAUSES OF CKD

- **Diabetes mellitus:** Most common cause of CKD due to high prevalence of disease.
- **Hypertension:** It can be cause as well as effect of CKD.
- Glomerulonephritis (inflammation of glomeruli).
- Interstitial nephritis (inflammation of tubulointerstitium compartment of kidneys)—various infections, autoimmune diseases and drugs can cause these diseases.
- Polycystic kidney disease like ADPKD or other inherited kidney diseases Alport syndrome.
- Obstruction of urinary tract (enlarged prostate, kidney stones and some cancers).
- Vesicoureteral reflux (back flow of urine into kidneys resulting in scarring).
- Recurrent kidney infection (pyelonephritis).

Complications

It include poor quality of life to life threatening complications:

- Fluid overload, including swelling of legs to pulmonary edema (fluid in lungs) which is life threatening emergency.

- Hyperkalemia which can leads to life-threatening heart block and cardiac arrest, need immediate treatment.
- Uremic encephalopathy which can cause difficulty concentrating, personality changes and seizures.
- Pericarditis (inflammation and fluid in pericardium) is urgent indication for starting dialysis.
- Anemia due to deficiency of erythropoietin (which is produced from kidney), iron deficiency, blood loss from intestine as well as in dialysis procedure, reduced blood formation due to inflammation.
- Heart disease and strokes due to fast atherosclerosis.
- **Mineral bone disease:** Weak bones and an increased risk of fractures occur due to PTH related poor quality bone formation.
- Decreased sex drive and erectile dysfunction.
- Decreased immunity leads to more infection.
- Pregnancy complications that carry risks for the mother and the developing fetus.

TREATMENT

- **Fluid overload:** This condition is treated with high dose of loop diuretics (furosemide and torsemide) or dialysis (hemodialysis, hemodiafiltration, and acute peritoneal dialysis), removing excess fluid. Fluid restriction is also advised.
- **Hyperkalemia:** This condition is treated with injectable calcium gluconate, dextrose with insulin infusion, asthalin nebulization, potassium-binding resins, and various modalities of dialysis.
- Uremic encephalopathy, pericarditis, and uremic symptoms are also treated with initiation of dialysis.
- **Correction of anemia:** Anemia is corrected with erythropoiesis-stimulating agents (ESA), iron therapy and blood transfusion. ESA stimulate the bone marrow to make red blood cells. The following types of ESAs (short acting ESA and long acting ESA) which are given SC are available erythropoietin(Epo), Epoetin alfa, Epoetin beta, Darbepoetin alfa, Methoxy polyethylene glycol-epoetin beta (Mircera). Short acting ESA are given once or twice a week and long acting ESA are given weekly or fortnightly. ESA are usually started when hemoglobin falls below 10 gm/dL and target Hb is 9–11.5 gm/dL. Over treatment with ESA to hemoglobin more than 13 gm/dL is associated with more number of strokes and heart attacks. Before starting ESA iron stores of body should be replenished by oral or parental iron. Usually 500–1,000 mg of iron is given by parental route depending on preparation type. Common iron preparation include iron dextrans, ferrous glauconite, iron sucrose, ferumoxytol and ferric carboxymaltose.
- **Hyperphosphatemia:** High phosphate are risk factor for cardiovascular cause of death. This condition is treated with calcium based and noncalcium-based phosphate binders like calcium acetate, calcium carbonate, sevelamer, ferric citrate, and lanthanum. Cinacalcet is also used in dialysis patients to lower phosphate levels.
- **Vitamin D deficiency and hypocalcemia:** This condition is treated with vitamin D and calcium supplements.
- **Antihypertensives:** CKD patients often require different classes of antihypertensive drugs to control blood pressure like calcium channel blockers, beta blockers, ACE inhibitors/angiotensin receptor blockers, diuretics, alpha antagonists, alpha2 adrenergic agonists, and others.

- **Vaccination:** CKD patients are often vaccinated for Hep B: 4 doses 1 mL intramuscular (IM) both deltoid at 0,1,2 and 6 months, Pneumococcal (Prevanar-13, 0.5 mL IM stat followed by Pneumovax 0.5 mL IM after 8 weeks and yearly influenza vaccine o.5 mL IM.
- **Renal replacement therapy (dialysis):** Dialysis is usually initiated when GFR falls to 7–8 mL/min/1.73 m^2 or even at little higher GFR when patients develop complications. Patients are given options of various forms of renal replacement therapy including renal transplant, hemodialysis and peritoneal dialysis. Patients can choose therapy as per their convenience and choice. Transplant is best form of therapy but is limited by organ availability. Hemodialysis is generally thrice in a week in center therapy lasting 4–5 hrs and procedure is carried out by dialysis nurse or technician. Potential issues with hemodialysis are access related and hemodynamic stress. Continuous ambulatory peritoneal dialysis (CAPD) is home-based therapy where patients are trained to continue 3–4 session of PD at home. It offer more independence and freedom and doesn't involve blood loss and access related issues, however CAPD peritonitis is major complication and can result in removal of catheter and discontinuation of therapy.
- Diet in CKD

Salt restriction (sodium <2 gm/day) is recommended in all stages of CKD. In pre dialysis patients protein restriction to 0.8 gm/kg/day is recommended, however, protein intake should be increased to 1.2 gm/kg/day in dialysis patients. Another strategy to prevent CKD progression is very low protein diet (0.55–0.6 gm/kg/day) along with keto acid analogues supplementation in pre dialysis patient. High potassium food (citrus fruits, banana, coconut water, sweet potatoes, spinach and packed bakery products) should be avoided in advanced CKD to prevent hyperkalemia. Phosphate rich processed food should also be restricted in advanced CKD.

SUGGESTED READING

1. Definition and classification of CKD. Kidney Int Suppl (2011). 2013;3(1):19-62.
2. Inker LA, Astor BC, Fox CH, Isakova T, Lash JP, Peralta CA, et al. KDOQI US commentary on the 2012 KDIGO clinical practice guideline for the evaluation and management of CKD. Am J Kidney Dis. 2014;63(5):713-35.
3. KDIGO. Clinical Practice Guideline for the Evaluation and Management of Chronic Kidney Disease 2012.

Hemodialysis: Basics and Principles

5
CHAPTER

Vijoy Kumar Jha, Arun Kumar S, Dipankar Bhowmik

INTRODUCTION

Dialysis involves passing the patient's blood against a semi-permeable membrane, with dialysis solution on the other side. Dialysis works on the broad principles of the movement of solutes and filtration of fluid across a semi-permeable membrane. The three principles that make dialysis work are diffusion, osmosis, and ultrafiltration, as shown in **Figure 1**.

DIFFUSION

It is the spontaneous movement of a solute from a solution with a higher solute concentration to a solution with a lower solute concentration across a semipermeable membrane. There is no movement of water in diffusion. A semipermeable membrane is a natural or synthetic membrane (for example, dialysis membrane) that allows certain ions and molecules to pass through very small openings (pores) present in them.

Diffusion in Dialysis

Dialysis means the diffusion of solutes across a semipermeable membrane down a concentration gradient with the greatest rate of diffusion when the concentration gradient is highest. It is the main mechanism for the removal of nitrogenous waste products and correcting the electrolyte, water, and acid-base abnormalities associated with renal failure. The use of a semipermeable membrane allows the passage of water and small molecular weight solutes but not large molecules like protein.

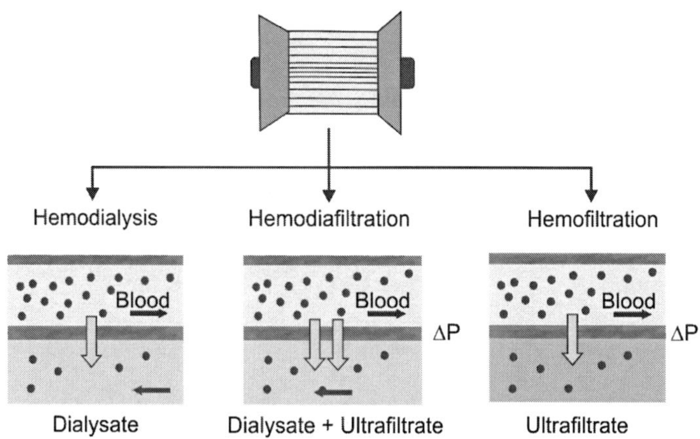

Fig. 1: Shows the principles of hemodialysis.

The temperature of the solution increases the rate of diffusion, while the viscosity and large molecules decrease the rate of diffusion. High flux membranes are thin with large pores and have a low resistance to diffusion. Only the free fraction of protein-bound solutes will be removed by diffusion.

Dialysis Concentrate and Dialysate

A concentrate is a mixture of treated water and chemicals mixed in the proper proportion and stored in a concentrated form. This concentrate is used for preparing the dialysis fluid (dialysate) by mixing the correct volume of the concentrate and treated water. The osmolality of dialysis fluid must be close to that of normal blood. The machines for bicarbonate dialysis have two mixing systems, one each for acid and bicarbonate concentrates. In the machine, mixing occurs in the proportion of acid concentrate: treated water: bicarbonate concentrate = 1:34:1.83.

What Happens in Dialysis?

In dialysis, blood and dialysate are pumped through two separate compartments separated by a semipermeable membrane. While the blood contains waste products of metabolism like urea, creatinine, etc., the dialysate solutions consist of purified water, sodium, potassium, magnesium, calcium, chloride, dextrose, and bicarbonate or acetate.

Diffusion of waste products (urea, creatinine, etc.) from blood to the dialysate compartment happens and is maximized by maintaining a high blood and dialysate flow rate, and also by pumping both these solutions (blood and dialysate) in opposite directions (countercurrent flow, as shown in **Figure 2**). By generating more Trans Membrane Pressure (TMP). Within the dialyser, more convective clearance can be added. Nowadays, it is automatically done in the volumetric UF controlled dialysis machines.

In conventional hemodialysis, small MW molecules are almost entirely cleared by diffusion. Large MW molecules (Beta 2 microglobulin or vitamin B12) are removed more effectively by convection which has led to increasing use of UF methods in hemodialysis as hemodiafiltration (HDF) or high volume hemofiltration. In continuous renal replacement therapy, convective mechanisms are mainly used for solute removal.

Molecular Cut-off

The molecular weight (MW) above which the substance will be unable to cross the membrane. MW is represented as Daltons. Most plasma proteins, RBC, WBC, and platelets are too large

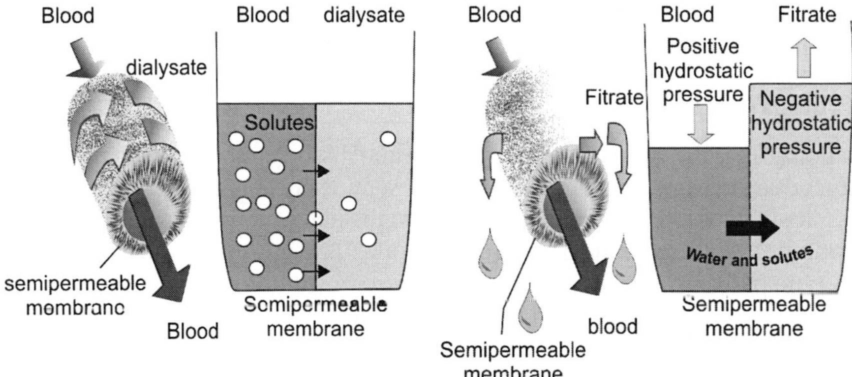

Fig. 2: Diffusion and ultrafiltration in dialysis.

to pass through dialysis membrane pores. High-cut-off membranes allow molecules up to 65,000 D to pass through them. Plasmapheresis membranes allow plasma with proteins and immunoglobulins to pass through with an MW cut-off of about 3,000 KD. The molecular weight of some common substances is—Urea (60D), Creatinine (113D), Glucose (184D), middle molecules (3,000–60,000 D), IgG (160,000 D), IgM (900,000 D), etc.

Clearance

It is the amount of blood that is completely cleared of a given solute in 1 min. Urea clearance of 200 mL/min at a blood flow rate of 300 mL/min means that the dialysis membrane should totally clear all the urea from 200 mL out of 300 mL of blood passing through it every minute.

Factors Affecting Solute Clearance

The amount of blood cleared of a given solute is the clearance (mL/min) and is measured from the reduction in blood urea concentration × blood flow rate. **Increasing the blood flow rate** increases the solute clearance but this increase is not proportional due to reduced diffusion efficiency. Most units aim blood flow rate of at least 250-35 mL/min. In practice, a 100% increase in blood flow rate increases urea clearance by only 20–50%. **Increasing dialysate flow rate** increases mild increase in clearance—an increase from 500 to 800 mL/min will increase urea clearance by no more than 10%. **Dialyser efficiency**—the pore size, membrane thickness, and architecture of the dialyser membrane affect solute clearance. KoA (mass transfer area coefficient) denotes the efficiency of solute clearance and KoA >800 mL/min is considered a high-efficiency dialyser. Switching to a higher KoA dialyser has a greater effect on small solute clearance compared to increasing blood or dialyser flow rate. Increasing the blood flow rate will be more effective in a high-efficiency dialyser. There is less effect on the clearance of large molecules on increasing blood flow rate as these molecules diffuse slowly. The duration of the dialysis session determines the effectiveness of solute clearance.

Efficiency of Dialysis

It depends on the urea clearance rate and KoA (mass transfer coefficient × surface area) of the dialyser. Urea clearance rate (>210 mL/min) and KoA (>800 mL/min) is considered high-efficiency dialyser. At a low blood flow rate (<200 mL/min), the advantage of a high-efficiency dialyser is not seen. Other than high KoA and high blood flow rate, high-efficiency dialysers require large surface area membranes, high dialysate flow, and bicarbonate dialysate. Increasing the solute clearance requires vascular access with good blood flow >200 mL/min along with higher dialysate flow (>500 mL/min). In conventional dialysis, the surface area varies from 0.5 to 1.3 m^2 with a larger surface area requirement for patients with higher body weight.

ULTRAFILTRATION (FILTRATION)

Ultrafiltration (UF) is the convective flow of water and dissolved solutes causing solvent drag of small solutes due to hydrostatic forces through the semipermeable membrane. In hemodialysis, it is the result of the negative pressure generated in the dialysate compartment by the dialysate effluent pump, i.e., transmembrane pressure (TMP). It is the pressure difference across the membrane between venous pressure (pressure in venous drip chamber) and dialysate (negative) pressure. The necessary TMP needed to remove a given volume of excess water can be calculated from the ultrafiltration coefficient (KUf) of the dialyser (provided by the manufacturer). KUF is the volume of fluid removed from blood in each hour for each mm

Hg pressure difference across the membranes, i.e., ultrafiltration in one hour = KUF X TMP. The dialysis membranes can be low or high-flux membranes differing in their permeability to water and solutes, being measured as the UF coefficient. The UF coefficient (KUf) can vary from 2 to 50 mL/h/mm Hg; >10 mL/h/mm Hg indicates high water permeability.

Ultrafiltration During Hemodialysis

Ultrafiltration is used to remove the excess water accumulated during dialysis sessions or to achieve adequate solute clearance by filtration (convection), as shown in **Figure 2**. For this online generation of ultrapure water or replacement fluids are required. UF provides better clearance of large MW solutes as compared to hemodialysis. Middle molecules of uremic toxins are better removed by this method of hemodiafiltration using high-flux membranes. Volumetric control is a much more accurate method of UF control, especially with the use of higher flux membranes. There are issues with errors in the measurement of TMP and changing KUF of dialysers during a dialysis session (due to protein deposition, partial blood clotting, and changes in hematocrit) which may cause significant volume changes. All modern dialysis machines with volumetric control systems measure the UF rate directly by quantifying the volume of dialysate after adjusting the flow rates.

High and Low Flux Dialysis

High flux dialyser refers to a high permeability membrane (beta 2 microglobulin clearance >20 mL/min) with better middle and large-molecule clearance. There is always a risk of back filtration from dialysate into blood and therefore, ultrapure pyrogen-free dialysate and bicarbonate buffering are required. Few small studies have suggested that high flux membranes may lead to better nutritional status and preservation of residual renal function but did not demonstrate any mortality benefit. In hemodiafiltration, dialysis with large volume UF is combined using high flux membranes performing convective and diffusive clearance of solutes.

HEMODIAFILTRATION

Hemodiafiltration is the simultaneous use of hemodialysis and ultrafiltration for water and solute clearance. In this mode, ultrapure replacement fluid, high flux membranes, high blood flow, good vascular access, and accurate volumetric control of UF replacement are very important. This procedure is widely accepted nowadays due to falling hemodiafilters prices and online production of pure replacement fluids from dialysate concentrates and water using two or three ultrafilters. Predilution replacement reduces the clearance and UF should be increased to deliver equivalent clearances. Postdilution replacement leads to hemoconcentration in the dialyser and protein fouling of the dialysis membrane. As inflammatory markers are improved, it may be especially useful for patients likely to be on dialysis for a long time. It may also be useful in those patients in whom it is difficult to achieve adequate Kt/V. Residual renal function is better preserved with HDF. UF volume of more than 21 L has improved mortality in observational studies.

Sieving Coefficient (SC)

The percentage of solute that passes through the membrane from the blood into the dialysate by convection. The convective transport of the solute depends on the SC of the membrane. SC is expressed from 0.1 to 1.0. SC of 0.4 means only 40% of solute passes through the membrane. The SC for larger molecules will be low in low-flux membranes and high in high-flux membranes.

Conductivity

The concentration of sodium in the dialysate prepared by the machine is denoted by the term "conductivity". The amount of electricity passing through the dialysate depends on the sodium concentration and the machine is programed to discard the dialysis fluid if the conductivity is beyond the permitted range. Newer machines can adjust the sodium concentration during dialysis sessions according to the set pattern, i.e., sodium profiling.

SUGGESTED READING

1. Chmielewski C, Filippone EJ. Principles and Practice of Dialysis. Nephrol Nurs J. 2004;31(3):349-50.
2. Henrich WL, editor. Principles and practice of dialysis. Lippincott Williams & Wilkins; 2009.
3. Luo J, Wu C, Xu T, Wu Y. Diffusion dialysis-concept, principle and applications. J Membrane Sci. 2011;366(1-2):1-6.

Hemodialysis Machine

6
CHAPTER

Sanjay Panda, KV Baliga, Sandeep Mahajan

OVERVIEW

The Hemodialysis (HD) machine is the functional element of the hemodialysis unit. Over the past decades, there have been improvements to the HD machine with introduction of newer technologies in terms of electronics, digitalization, and miniaturization. However, the basic principles of the HD machine have remained the same. For understanding hemodialysis therapy, it is important to understand the mechanism of HD machine.

DEFINITION

The hemodialysis machine is defined as a mixing device with a blood pump to propel the blood through an extracorporeal circuit (hollow fiber membrane and tubing). The basic aim being to bring the dialysate in contact with the blood across a semipermeable membrane (dialyser) for the process of diffusion and convection to take place **(Fig. 1)**. The primary role of the machine is to prepare the dialysate by mixing treated water with acid and bicarbonate concentrate. The machine delivers the dialysate in a countercurrent direction relative to direction of blood flow across the dialyser membrane **(Fig. 2)**. The HD machine is divided into three parts:

1. Fluid delivery system with its monitors and control panel **(Fig. 1)**.
2. Blood circuit with its monitors and control panel **(Fig. 2)**.
3. Electrical systems

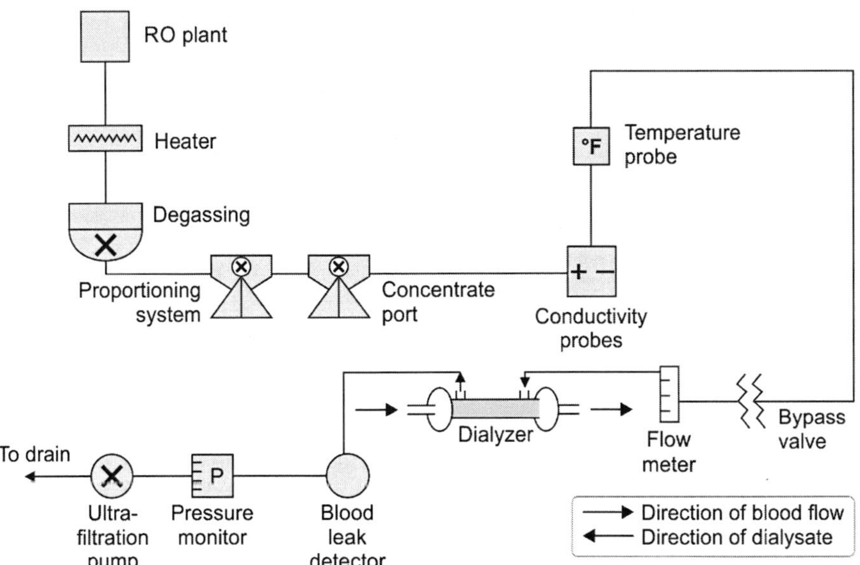

Fig. 1: Flowchart of dialysate flow.
(*Courtesy:* Pihord J Hemodialysis Training Manual, 7th edition)

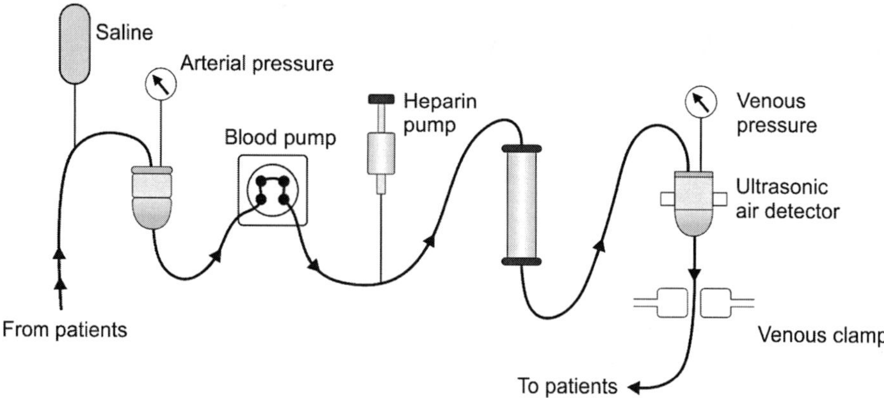

Fig. 2: Blood circuit.
(*Courtesy:* Pihord J Hemodialysis Training Manual, 7th edition)

DIALYSATE SOLUTION

The dialysate is an aqueous nonsterile fluid with level of electrolytes equivalent to extracellular fluid with exceptions of lower potassium and higher bicarbonate levels. The solution is isotonic with an osmolarity of 300 +/– 10 mosmol/L. The solution contains six electrolyte components (sodium, potassium, calcium, magnesium, chloride and bicarbonate) and one nonelectrolyte component namely dextrose (100–200 mg /L). The potassium concentration in the dialysate is usually 2.5 mEq/L and the bicarbonate concentration is 30–35 mEq/L. The dialysate is freshly prepared and makes one pass through the dialyser to maintain an even concentration gradient across the dialyser membrane.

FLUID DELIVERY SYSTEM

Majority of the dialysis centers use HD machines which are self-contained for the preparation of the dialysate. The dialysate is prepared in the machine itself.

Dialysate Circuit Components

Water Inlet Solenoid Valve

The treated water from the reverse osmosis plant flows into the dialysis machine through a water inlet solenoid valve when the machine is switched on and stops when the machine is switched off. The valve permits the entry of treated water at a pressure between 20 and 105 psi (pounds per square inch). The process is important to prevent water logging when the machine is switched off. This prevents bacterial contamination if water is stagnant in the machine. A manometer measures the inlet pressure. Inadequate flow or pressure will lead to a continuous audible alarm **(Figs. 3 and 4)**.

Dialysate Heater

A heater system raises the temperature on incoming water. The process partially degasses the water and improves the mixing qualities of the water with the concentrate. The heating temperature is controlled by thermistor feedback circuit. The dialysis machine is provided with a fine adjustment knob on the control panel. The dialysate temperature is maintained between 37 and 38°C. The machine has a low and high temperature alarm. In case the preset limits are

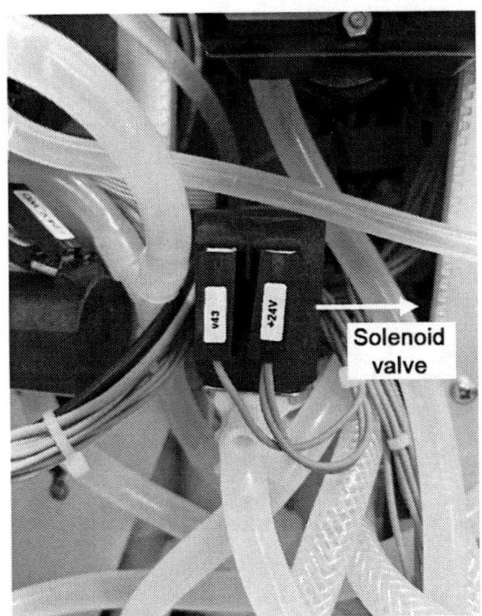

Fig. 3: Solenoid valve.
(*Courtesy:* Fresenius Medical Care, India)

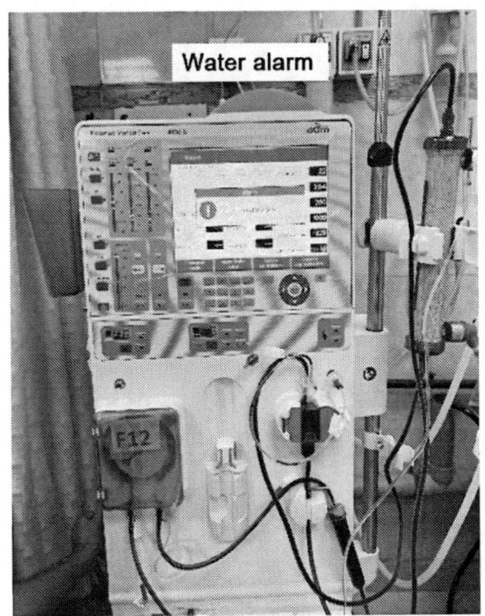

Fig. 4: Water alarm.
(*Courtesy:* Fresenius Medical Care, India)

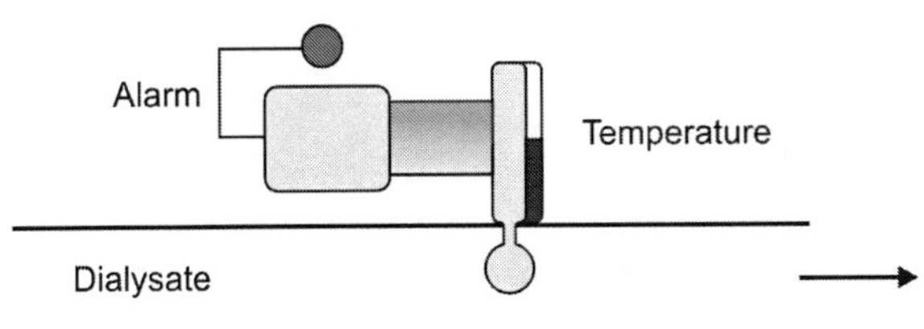

Fig. 5: Dialysate temperature monitor.
(*Courtesy:* Pihord J Hemodialysis Training Manual, 7th edition)

exceeded, the machine is designed to give an audio alarm, a visual alarm, and go into bypass mode (dialysate flow is stopped). The function of bypass valve is described ahead **(Figs. 5 and 6).**

Deaeration System

The system consists of a vacuum pump which exposes the treated water to subatmospheric pressure resulting in removal of dissolved gases. The gases form bubbles are vented to atmosphere by a bubble trap in the machine. The removal of gases from the treated water is an important function to improve the efficacy of dialysis and prevent microbubbles from enter, circulation, leading to air embolism. Rapid fluctuations in conductivity (described ahead) or frequent blood leak alarms indicate a malfunction of the vacuum pump **(Fig. 7)**.

Mixing Device

The device proportionates treated water and dialysate concentrate (acid and bicarbonate) to create a dialysate with correct ionic concentration. The mixing ratios of water to dialysate concentration are:

- 34:1–44:1 for acid concentrate
- 20:1–25:1 for bicarbonate concentrate

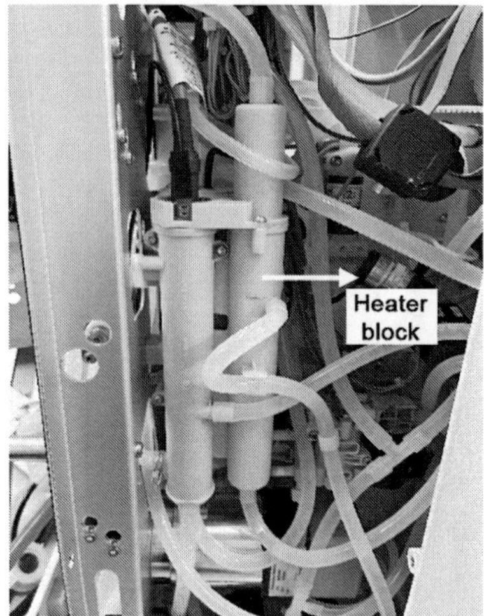

Fig. 6: Heater block.
(*Courtesy:* Fresenius Medical Care, India)

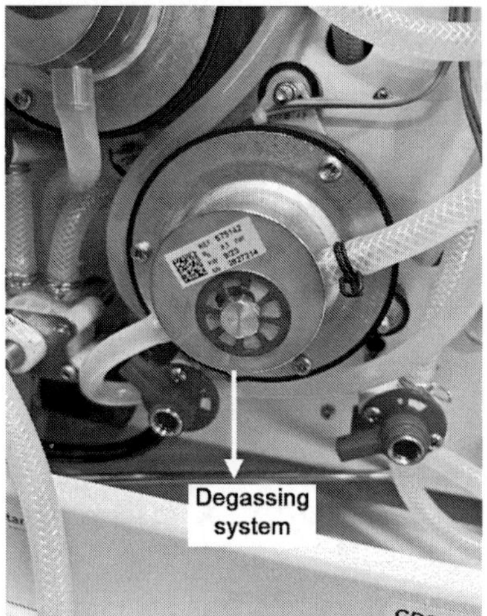

Fig. 7: Degassing system.
(*Courtesy:* Fresenius Medical Care, India)

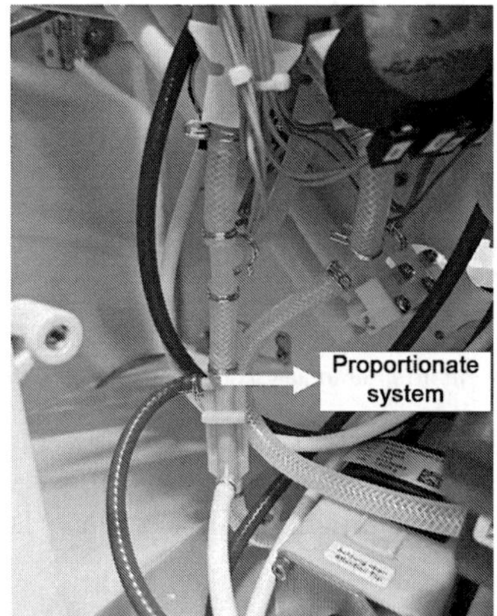

Fig. 8: Proportionating system.
(*Courtesy:* Fresenius Medical Care, India)

The mixing device is servo controlled and continuously adjusts the dialysate concentrates till the conductivity sensors reach the desired conductivity. The working of mixing device is monitored by conductivity and pH monitors. There are two conductivity monitors in an HD machine. Careful checks should be done for putting the acid and bicarbonate concentrates to the correct ports as reversal of ports could expose the patient to a lethal ionic concentration as the respective pumps are fixed at different fixed ratios **(Fig. 8)**.

Conductivity Monitors

The conductivity is measured by a two-electrode system. The electrodes are connected to a constant current device and an ammeter. The conductivity cell is made of corrosion resistant material and is connected to a meter that displays the reading of total ionic concentration on

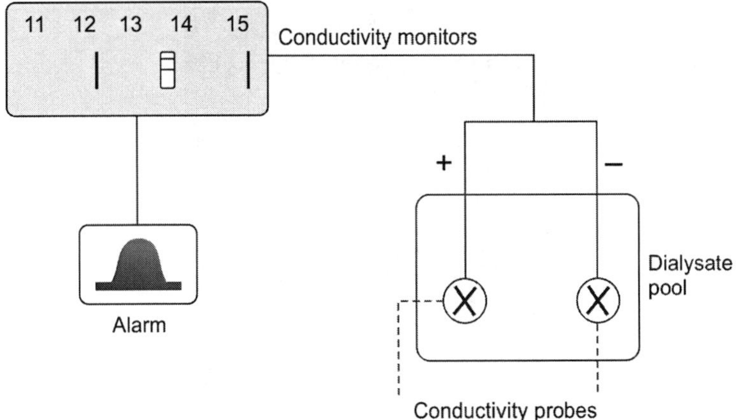

Fig. 9: Conductivity monitor.
(*Courtesy:* Pihord J Hemodialysis Training Manual, 7th edition)

the front panel. The conductivity meter reads the conductivity in millimhos per centimeter (nmos/cm). The acceptable range is between 12.5 and 16.0 mmhos/cm. The two conductivity monitoring cells maintain a double redundancy. The cell activate high-low alarms at different limits of internal tolerance. The first set of conductivity cells is activated at +/– 5% and the second set of cells is at +/– 50% of normal conductivity. Unless the HD machine achieves the set level of conductivity, it will not start dialysis. Once a conductivity alarm goes on, the following actions are taken by the machine, an audible alarm, a visual alarm and the machine goes into bypass mode diverting the dialysate to the drain. No change in conductivity setting should be done while the patient is on dialysis. Low conductivity alarm is usually due to lack of either acid or bicarbonate concentrate or incorrect dialysate ionic concentration. High conductivity alarm is due to inadequate water flow, water with high calcium content or incorrect connections of the acid or bicarbonate concentrates into the wrong ports **(Figs. 9 and 10)**.

pH Control

Newer model HD machines are fitted with an inbuilt pH sensor and will not go into conductivity testing till pH of dialysate is 7.5 +/– 0.5.

Bypass System

The valve directs the dialysate to the drain instead of the dialyser and is activated by high/low conductivity, high/low pH or high/low temperature of the dialysate **(Fig. 11)**.

Rinse Function

This function overrides the bypass valve and should not be activated while the patient is on dialysis. However, as a built-in safety feature, the blood pump stops on activation of the rinse mode.

Dialysate Pressure Monitor and Volumetric Control

This function of the machine ensures safe and exact fluid removal. The method employed is to generate a transmembrane pressure (TMP) to generate ultrafiltrate **(Fig. 1)**. The machine has a volumetric control system-based on balancing chamber to measure the fluids entering and leaving the dialyser. By setting an ultrafiltrate goal, the software of the machine automatically

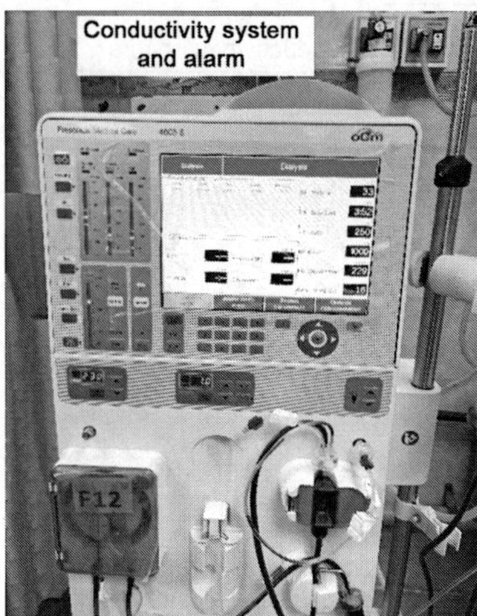

Fig. 10: Conductivity alarm.
(*Courtesy:* Fresenius Medical Care, India)

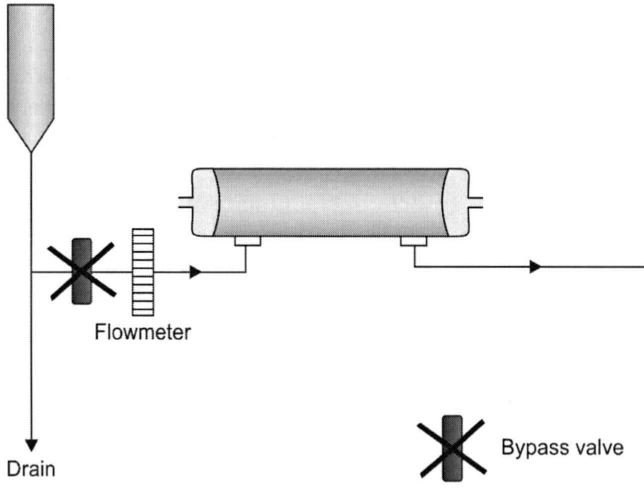

Fig. 11: Bypass valve.
(*Courtesy:* Pihord J Hemodialysis Training Manual, 7th edition)

adjusts the transmembrane pressure. The volumetric control uses matched pumps controlled by valves and integrated after the dialysate has undergone proportioning. These valves placed above and below the balancing chamber open and close sequentially, pushing as well as removing dialysate into the drain. There are two sets of balancing chambers which work alternatingly ensuring a constant supply of dialysate. The whole system works in a closed loop. Air is removed from the dialysate via an auxiliary vacuum pump to ensure accurate measurement. Pressure holding test for the balancing systems are performed automatically by the machine prior to initiation of dialysis.

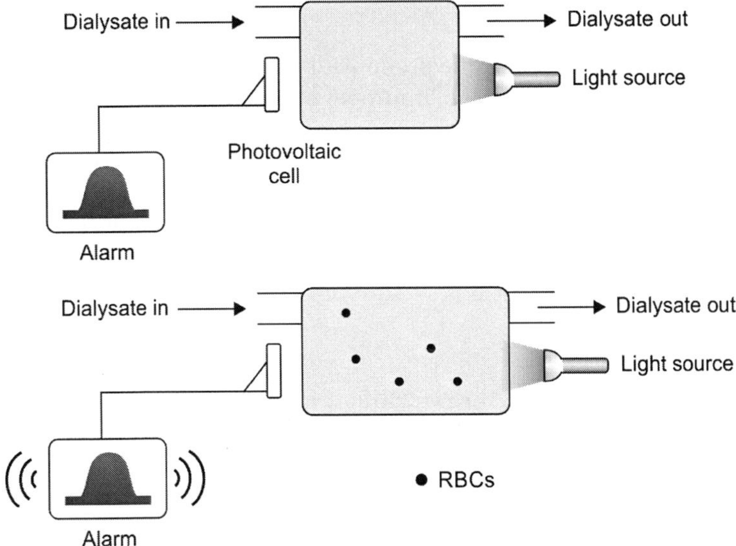

Fig. 12: Blood leak detector system.
(*Courtesy:* Pihord J Hemodialysis Training Manual, 7th edition)

Blood Leak Detector System

The system works on the principle of transmission of light through a column of effluent. In case of a tear in dialyser membrane the photovoltaic cell does not receive the light from the source and triggers an audible and visual alarm. The threshold for the detection system is set at 0.25–0.35 mL of whole blood. False alarms are caused by air bubbles or dirt in the optical system **(Fig. 12)**.

Dialysate Flow

The dialysate depending on the machine is preset or adjustable and the range for conventional dialysis is 500 mL/min while for high-efficiency dialysis, it is 800 mL/min. The dialysate flow is usually one- and -a-half times the blood flow rate. In case of low incoming water pressure, dialysate pump failure or flow path obstruction, a continuous audible alarm is initiated.

Effluent Line

The dialysate effluent line should be placed into a drain in a unobstructed manner as obstruction can produce back pressure and decrease dialysate flow.

BLOOD CIRCUIT

The blood pump propels the blood into the extracorporeal circuit (dialyser and tubing) and has monitors for arterial and venous line pressure monitoring. The arterial line is the access for blood from the patient to the blood pump. It can be a temporary catheter (red color coded), permanent catheter (red color coded), arteriovenous fistula or arteriovenous graft. The return of blood from the dialyser is through the venous line (blue coded) to the catheters (blue coded), arteriovenous fistulas or arteriovenous graft. The circuit is also equipped with air detectors and blood leak detector (described above) **(Fig. 12)**.

Blood Pump

The blood pump is a rotatory peristaltic pump with rollers on which the tubing is mounted. The pump requires adequate calibration. Improper tubing with narrowing or occlusion due to improper mounting can be a potential cause for blood leaks and hemolysis. The blood pump has an on-off switch. The flow rate can be varied from 50 mL/min to 500 mL/min which can be regulated from the front panel. The stoppage of blood pump during dialysis triggers an audible and visual alarm. The blood pump is also connected to the blood leak detector and as a safety feature the machine shuts down in case of a blood leak alarm. Usual flow rates are between 200 mL/min and 400 mL/min **(Fig. 12)**.

Arterial Pressure Monitor

The pressure monitor in the machine is connected to the tubing via a sterile transducer which accesses the prepump arterial drip chamber via an extension line in the tubing. This portion of the circuit is venerable to air leaks and the transducer is essential to prevent viral contamination. The pressure monitors should be open during dialysis and the high-low limits should be set in the range of 50 to 100 mm of Hg. The arterial pressure monitor is leak-free and reads negative and positive pressure and the limits are open during set-up, priming and rinsing. The dialysis personnel must set the low negative pressure reading below the value on start of therapy. The low-pressure alarm is triggered by hypotension, kink in the arterial line, clot in the arterial line or malposition of access device. The high-pressure alarm is triggered by leaking and torn tubing in prepump segment, saline infusion line being unclamped, increase in patient's blood pressure. The activation of the alarms results in an audible alarm, stoppage of the blood pump and the control panel shows arterial pressure readings to be out of range. The actions which need to be taken are mute the alarm, identify the problem, correct it and restart the blood pump.

Venous Pressure Monitor

This device monitors postpump pressure in the extracorporeal circuit and is connected to the machine via a line attached to the postpump drip chamber and hooked to the manometer in the machine via a transducer. The transducer has the same function as the arterial line transducer and are identical single use devices. The limits of the venous circuit are set between - 50 mm of Hg and + 150 mm of Hg. The cause of high-pressure alarm is usually a kink in the venous line, clots in the drip chamber or venous access device malposition or occlusion. The cause of low-pressure alarm is venous line separation from the access device, leak in the tubing, dialyser leak, dialyser clotting and a very low blood pump speed. The venous pressure determines the transmembrane pressure and the ultrafiltration rate via the equation, that is; $TMP = P_{\text{Blood line}} - P_{\text{Dialysate line}}$.

Therefore, high venous pressure can increase ultrafiltration. The venous pressure alarm results in an audible sound, a visual reading on the front panel of the machine and stoppage of the blood pump. The problem should be identified and fixed before the pump is restarted. The sequence is the same as for arterial alarm **(Figs. 2 and 16)**.

Air-foam Detector

They are ultrasonic devices which are clamped to the venous line following its exit from the venous drip chamber. They are designed to detect air bubbles in the range of 50–500 microns. The prepump circuit has a negative pressure and the postpump circuit has a positive pressure.

The air-foam detector should be checked periodically. The activation of air-foam sets up an audible alarm, stops the blood pump and engages the venous clamp. The problem rectification should include examination of venous drip chamber for foam, drop in level of arterial drip chamber, foam in arterial drip chamber and foam in venous line. The problem should be identified and rectified prior to disengagement of the clamp and re-start of the blood pump. The rectification measures include removal of foam in the circuit, filling up the venous chamber with saline or changing the blood lines prior to continuation of dialysis **(Figs. 13 and 14)**.

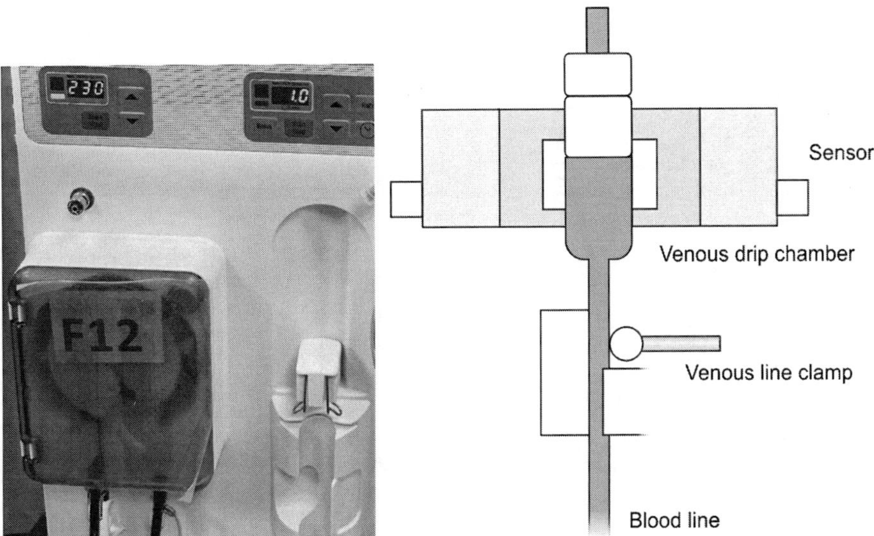

Fig. 13: Air detector system.
(*Courtesy:* Pihord J Hemodialysis Training Manual, 7th edition)

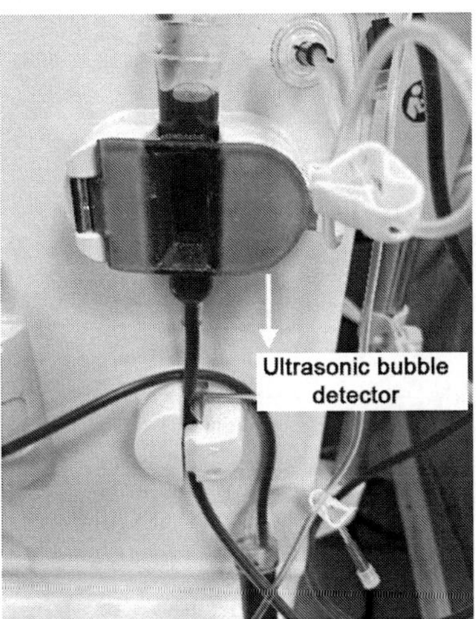

Fig. 14: Ultrasonic air-foam detector.
(*Courtesy:* Fresenius Medical Care, India)

Venous Line Clamp

This is an occlusive clamp located just below the ultrasonic air-foam detector. The clamp is designed to withstand a pressure gradient of 800 mm of Hg. The dialysis therapy should not be carried out without activation of air-foam detector and venous line clamp **(Figs. 15 and 16)**.

Heparin Infusion Pump

This is an electric-driven piston pump located on the postdialyser circuit and can be preset to deliver a bolus as well as hourly dosage of heparin infusion. The pump can be safely overridden but careful monitoring for dialyser clotting is required **(Fig. 17)**.

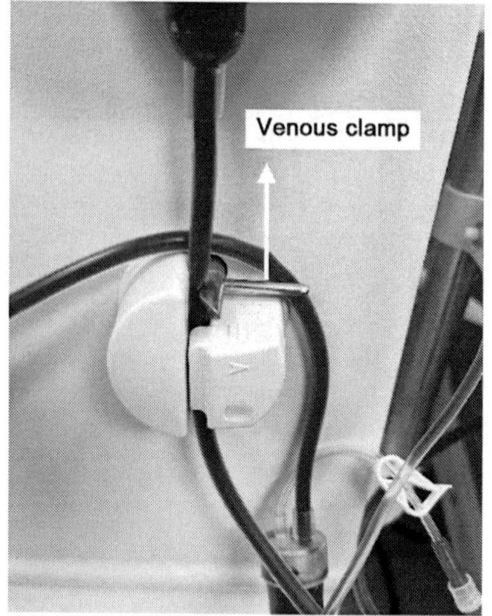

Fig. 15: Venous line clamp.
(*Courtesy:* Fresenius Medical Care, India)

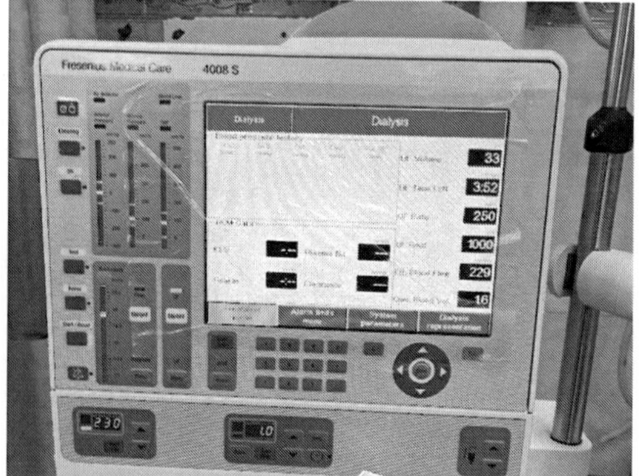

Fig. 16: Front panel display. Arterial and venous pressure monitor.
(*Courtesy:* Fresenius Medical Care, India)

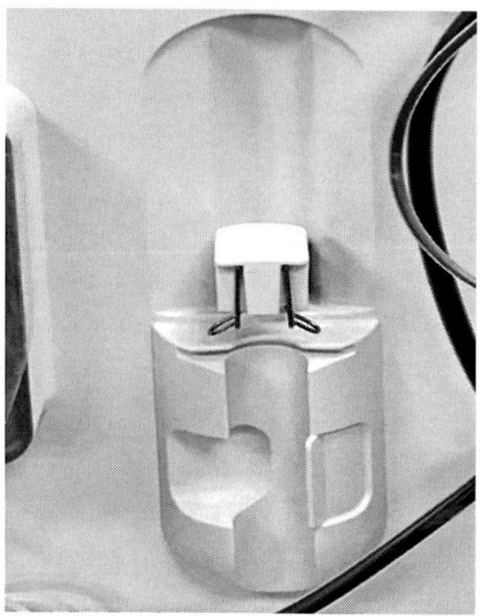

Fig. 17: Heparin pump.
(*Courtesy:* Fresenius Medical Care, India)

ELECTRONIC SYSTEMS AND SAFETY

The HD machine has a microprocessor-based motherboard which integrates the various pumps and monitors as well as the multiple feedback loops which activate the various safety features. This is the brain of the machine and is highly sensitive to voltage fluctuations. Damage to the motherboard will render the machine unsuitable to use. The dialysis machine can deliver a shock or get short-circuited and hence should be checked periodically for liquid leaks and proper earthing. The machine should have a proper socket connected to uniform power source. Electrical safety classes and safe use protocols are mandatory for all personnel using the machine.

The hemodialysis machine is a complex electromedical device-based on microprocessor-based technology with digital-analog interface. Although the principle of working is simple, the working elements needed to get the process completed are complex and need high degree of engineering expertise. A knowledge of the working principles of the machine is important both for patient and personnel safety.

SUGGESTED READING

1. Azar AT, Canaud B. Hemodialysis system. Volume 1: Techniques of Hemodialysis Systems. 2013:99-166.
2. Daschner M, Schaefer FS. Technical aspects of the hemodialysis procedure. In: Warady BA, Schaefer FS, Fine RN, Alexander SR (Eds). Dialysis. Springer, Dordrecht; 2004.
3. Selection and Use of Machine, Dialyser and Dialysis Fluid for Maintenance Hemodialysis. Indian J Nephrol. 2020;30(Suppl 1):S9-S17.

Dialyser

7
CHAPTER

Amit Katyal, Mehak Singla, PP Varma

INTRODUCTION

The dialyser is popularly called artificial kidney. It is a selective filter used for removing toxic or unwanted solutes from the blood. The filtration process uses a semipermeable membrane between blood flowing on one side and dialysis fluid, called dialysate, on the opposite side. The dialyser and the membrane constitute the heart, of renal replacement therapy.

COMPONENTS DIALYSER (FIG. 1)

- Blood compartment
- Dialysate compartment
- Semipermeable membrane
- Membrane support structure

Structure

In the hollow-fiber dialyser, the blood flows into a chamber at one end of the cylindrical shell called a header. From there, blood enters thousands of small capillaries tightly bound in a bundle. The dialyser is designed in such a way that blood flows through the fibers and dialysis solution flows around them in counter cloackwise fashion **(Fig. 1)**. Once through the capillaries, the blood collects in a header at the other end of the cylindrical shell and is then routed back to the patient through the venous tubing and venous access device.

TYPES OF DIALYSER (TABLE 1)

All dialysers consist of a series of parallel flow paths designed to provide a large surface area between blood and membrane, and membrane and dialysate. There are two basic flow path geometries—(1) rectangular cross section, seen in parallel plate dialysers and (2) circular cross section, seen in hollow-fiber dialysers. Virtually all hemodialysers in clinical use today are the hollow-fiber type. However, for historical purposes, the parallel plate and coil dialysers will be discussed.

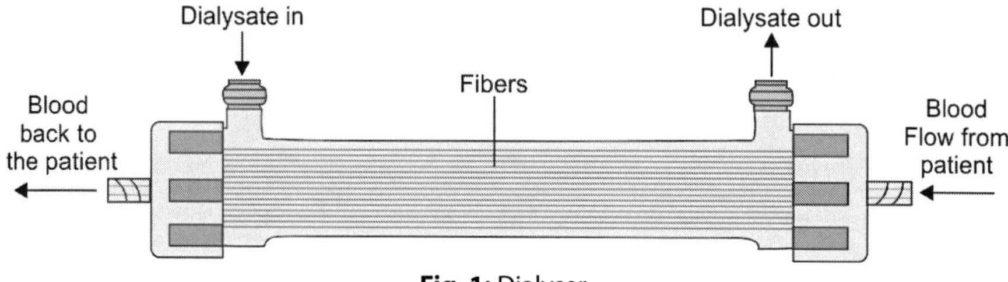

Fig. 1: Dialyser.

Table 1: Types of dialyser.

Types of dialyser	*Advantage*	*Disadvantages*
1. Coil dialyser	Easily available	• Large priming volume • UF unpredictable • Blood leaks common
2. Parallel plate	Low heparin requirement	• TMP increases the blood volume in the dialyser • Not suited for reuse
3. Hollow fiber	• Low heparin requirement • Reusable • TMP does not increases the blood volume in the dialyser	

Coil Dialysers

These consisted of a cellulose acetate membrane tightly wrapped around a plastic or metal coil, and encased in a rigid plastic housing. The priming volume was very large, ultrafiltration was unpredictable, and blood leaks were quite common.

Parallel Plate Dialysers

These are assembled in layers. Sheets of membrane were placed between supporting to support the membrane and allow the flow of dialysate along it. The blood flows through the sheets of the membrane. The contained volume of blood is small, and heparin requirements are also usually small. The main disadvantages is that the volume of blood that they hold increases as the transmembrane pressure (TMP) increases and are not well suited for reuse.

The Hollow-fiber Dialyser

This is by far the most commonly used dialyser and is available in various configurations. There are thousands of tiny hollow fibers of about 150–250 μm diameter. Blood flows through these hollow fibers. They are formed from a variety of materials, both cellulose and synthetic. Wall thickness may be as little as 7 μm, 50 μm or more. The contained blood volume is very low in relation to the dialyser's surface area because of the dialyser's flow geometry. Resistance to blood flow is low because of the large number of blood passages. Hollow-fiber dialysers are not compliant and hence they do not increase in shape or in the volume they hold under high TMP. Ultrafiltration can be precisely controlled. They are well adapted to reuse. Meticulous deaeration of the fiber bundle is required before beginning a dialysis procedure otherwise fibers may air lock and not admit blood. There may be uneven distribution of blood at the inflow header space, with reduced perfusion of some of the center fibers. Hollow-fiber dialysers may be sterilized with ethylene oxide (ETO). Residual toxic products of ETO sterilization retained in the potting material of the headers can cause adverse reactions.

DIALYSER MEMBRANES

Membranes are of two basic types:

1. Unsubstituted cellulose membranes
2. Substituted cellulose membranes
3. Synthetic membranes.

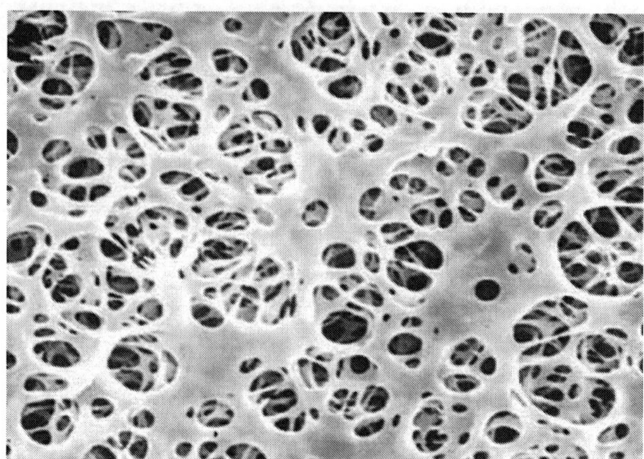

Fig. 2: Cellulose membrane.

Unsubstituted cellulose Membranes (Fig. 2)

Purified cellulose (e.g., from cotton linters) is dissolved in an ammoniac solution of cupric oxide and the cellulose polymer chain are newly arranged during the subsequent spinning process. The macroscopically homogenous membrane that is extremely hydrophilic, absorbs water and forms a hydrogel. Diffusion of solutes actually takes place through water-swollen regions rather than pores as observed for synthetic membranes. Due to their small membrane wall thickness, membranes made from regenerated cellulose have good diffusive low molecular weight clearances properties. In a well-designed dialyser, these clearances may be comparable, or even superior, to those of some low flux synthetic membranes. Disadvantages are the poor biocompatibility.

Substituted Cellulose Membranes

Developed via chemical modification to improve biocompatibility by replacing hydroxyl groups with acetate groups, such as cellulose acetate, cellulose diacetate (CDA), cellulose triacetate (CTA). These membranes lead to comparatively lower complement activation and can be sterilized by all common sterilization procedures (ETO, g-irradiation, steam).

Synthetic Membranes

The synthetic membranes are thermoplastics. They have a thin, smooth luminal surface supported by a sponge like wall structure. Those used for hemodialysis include polyacrylonitrile (PAN), polysulfone (PS) **(Fig. 3)**, polyamide, polymethyl methacrylate (PMMA), and others. Synthetic membranes have much fewer biocompatibility problems than cellulose membranes. Synthetic membranes were developed in the search for efficient ultrafiltration. They, in turn, have made high-flux hemodialysis, hemofiltration, and continuous renal replacement therapy viable options in renal treatment.

Membrane Performance

This depends on the pore size, surface area, membrane thickness, pore density and protein adsorption. High performance membranes have excellent biocompatibility, effective clearance of target solutes and larger pore size than conventional hemodialysis membranes promoting removal of middle to large molecular weight solutes including B2 microglobulin.

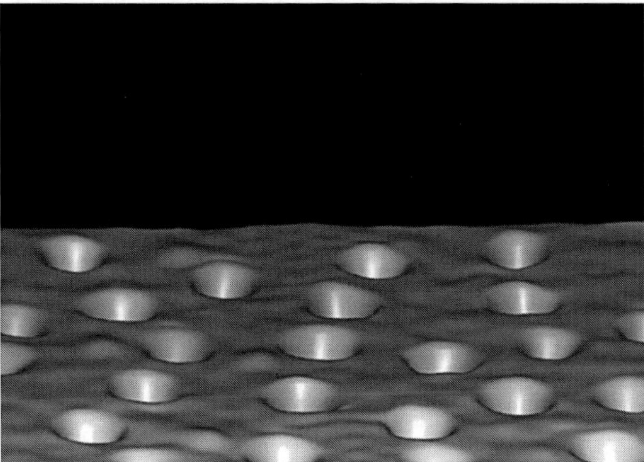

Fig. 3: Polysulfone membrane.

Membrane Biocompatibility

Each time blood comes in contact with a foreign surface, an inflammatory response is elicited. This response is used to gauge the biocompatibility of a hemodialysis membrane. When there is an intense reaction and a high level of inflammation, the membrane is said to be biocompatible. Biocompatibility can occur due to protein membrane interaction, complement and leukocyte activation and leaching and palliation. Cellulose membranes have free hydroxyl radicles in their structure. Complement in blood binds to these sites and gets activated with resultant leukocyte infiltration. Synthetic membranes lack the reactive sites found on cellulose-based membranes; thus the amount of complement activation generated during hemodialysis is less than with cellulose membranes. Long-term use of biocompatible membranes may be associated with an increased incidence of infection and malignancy and with impaired nutritional status.

DIALYSER PERFORMANCE

The various parameters used for performance are:

- **Clearance:** This is defined as the volume completely cleared of a given solute per unit time expressed in mL per minute. The in vivo clearance is lower than the in vitro clearance reported by the manufactures. KDOQI recommends target single pool Kt/V (spKt/V) of 1.4 per hemodialysis session for patient treated thrice weekly, with minimum delivered spKt/V of 1.2.
- **Mass transfer area coefficient:** Product of clearance of a solute and the surface area. Dialyser efficiency is primarily the ability of dialyser to remove small solutes. Dialysers can be low efficiency (K0A<500 mL/min) or high efficiency (K0A>600 mL/min).
- **Ultra filtration coefficient:** It is the permeability of dialyser to water expressed as Kuf (mL/h/mm Hg).
- **Flux of a dialyser:** It refers to the ability of a dialyser to remove very large molecules, such as beta 2 microglobulin.
- **Low flux dialysers:** Defined as beta 2 microglobulin clearance of <10 mL/mt and ultrafiltration rate <15 mL/mm Hg/Hr. They effectively remove small solutes through diffusion and only negligible amounts of middle molecules, e.g., FX 5/8/10.
- **High flux dialysers:** Defined as beta 2 microglobulin clearance of >20 mL/mt and Kuf of >15 mL/mm Hg/hr. Patients on long term dialysis have better survival outcomes with high flux vs low flux dialysers, e.g., FX60/80/100.

- **Protein Leaking Dialysers:** Japanese use protein leaking dialysers which not only remove middle molecules but some large molecule toxins also. This is how more or less glomerulus functions. Those protein leaking dialysers are recommended where albumin loss is not more than 3 g per session. Over 90% of Japanese dialysis population uses these type of dialysers.
- **Paed dialyser:** The volume of the extracorporeal blood circuit should not exceed 10% of the patient's blood volume. The best choice is a low flux dialyser. However newer HDF systems like 5,008 CorDiax Paed therapy can be used for 10 kg pediatric population. However if high flux dialysis is used therapy time should be reduced. Common pediatric dialysers are enumerated below.

Dialyser	*Membrane*	*Surface area*	*Prime volume (mL)*
Polyflux 6H	Polysulfone	0.6	52
F3+	Polysulfone	0.4	28
FX paed+	Helixone	0.2	18

DIALYSER REUSE

The use of the same dialyser for more than one therapy. Germicides like peracetic acid are instilled for disinfection. Though single use is the best option but if reuse is required for economic reasons than KDOQI recommends reuse only if fiber volume is minimum of 80% or urea clearance is 90% of original.

Advantages

- Reduces incidence of 'first use' dialyser reactions.
- Cost effective.

Disadvantage

If the reuse procedure is not thorough then adverse reactions as well as inadequate clearance can occur.

Reprocessing

The reprocessing can be manual or automated. The following procedure is followed for dialyser reprocessing prior to reuse:
- Cleaning and rinsing of the dialyser.
- Inspection to see for any broken fibers or blood leaks. If fiber volume is less than 80%, dialyser needs to be discarded.
- The dialyser is filled with a germicide properly labeled and stored. Before reuse, dialyser is tested to ensure no germicide is left.
- Dialyser should be tested prior to reuse.

Priming

The priming is an essential step in initiation of dialysis to prevent incidence of anaphylactic reactions by leachable agents. A new dialyser should be primed with 1 liter of saline and reprocessed dialyser by 2 liters of saline.

Recommendation for Dialyser Use

- It is recommended to use biocompatible, synthetic or modified cellulose membranes, to avoid reactions.

- Hemo Study and MPO trial found no benefit in mortality between high flux or low flux membranes. Patients who are diabetic or have serum albumin <4 g/dL or are on dialysis for longer duration of time may benefit from high-flux dialyser.
- KDOQI recommended the use of biocompatible, either high or low flux hemodialysis membranes for intermittent hemodialysis.
- Surface area of the dialyser should be chosen based on the required dialysis dose and the body size of the patient, so that single use KT/V of 1.4 is achieved.
- Japanese study and some other studies show that protein leaking or high flux dialysers have survival advantage, as they can remove middle molecules and some large sized solutes also.

SUGGESTED READING

1. Abe M, Masakane I, Wada A, Nakai S, Nitta K, Nakamoto H. Dialyzer Classification and Mortality in Hemodialysis Patients: A 3-Year Nationwide Cohort Study. Front Med (Lausanne). 2021;8:740461.
2. Bouré T, Vanholder R. Which dialyser membrane to choose? Nephrology Dialysis Transplantation. 2004;19(2):293-6.
3. Eknoyan G, Beck GJ, Cheung AK, et al. Effect of dialysis dose and membrane flux in maintenance hemodialysis. New Engl J Med. 2002;347:2010-9.
4. National Kidney Foundation. KDOQI Clinical Practice Guideline for Hemodialysis Adequacy: 2015 update. Am J Kidney Dis. 2015;66(5):884-930.
5. Uhlenbusch-Körwer I, Bonnie-Schorn E, Grassmann A, Vienken J: Understanding Membranes and Dialysers.

Dialysate

8

CHAPTER

Amit Katyal, Nikesh Agrawal, Vinant Bhargava

INTRODUCTION

Dialysate fluid can be considered a drug and is made by mixing two concentrate components, which may be provided in a liquid or dry forms. It is a non sterile solution that is similar to the normal level of electrolytes found in the extracellular fluid with the exception of potassium and bicarbonate. The dialysis machine has pumps and one-way valve systems that make the final dialysis solution by taking fixed volumes of dialysate concentrates and mixing them with a fixed volume of heated purified water, or by using conductivity-based servo control systems to mix the concentrates and water. The ionic composition of the final dialysis solution is checked by conductivity, which is kept in a very tight range with inbuilt alarm systems. If conductivity gets outside the range, an alarm sounds and dialysis stops.

DIALYSATE SOLUTION

It is almost an isotonic solution with range from 300 ± 20 milliosmoles per liter and is kept as close to the plasma osmolality. The commonly used components in the dialysis fluid are enumerated below:

Electrolyte	*Dialysate range*	*Blood level*
Na	135–145 mEq/L	135–145 mEq/L
K	0–4	3.5–5.5
Ca	2.25–3.0	4.5–5.5
Mg	0.5–1.0	1.5–2.5
Cl	100–115	95–105
HCO_3	30–40	22–28
Dextrose	0–200 mg/dl	80–120 mg/dL

Dialysate Sodium

With the advent of high clearance dialysers and more efficient dialysis techniques, the decline in plasma osmolality becomes more apparent as solute is more rapidly removed. Use of a high dialysate Na by preventing a decrease in plasma osmolality, led to mobilization of fluid from the intracellular space resulting in better preservation of plasma volume. The primary concern of high Na is in stimulating thirst and causing increased weight gain and poor blood pressure control. Varying the concentration of Na in the dialysate during the procedure can obviate this. A high dialysate Na concentration is used initially with a progressive reduction toward isotonic or hypotonic levels by the end of the procedure. This method allows for a diffusive Na influx early in the session to prevent the rapid decline in plasma osmolality resulting from the efflux of urea and other small molecular weight solutes. During the remainder of the procedure, when the reduction in osmolality accompanying urea removal is less abrupt, the lower dialysate Na level minimizes the development of hypertonicity and any resultant excessive thirst, fluid gain, and hypertension in the interdialytic period. However, this strategy is not data validated conclusively. In some patients a high/low Na protocol can lead to large interdialytic weight gain or cause intradialytic hypertension and hence the therapy needs to be individualized.

In hypertensive patients, the intradialytic sodium may be reduced to avoid hypertensive episodes, while in hypotensive patients increasing the dialysate sodium can favorably increase blood pressure and reduce symptoms like cramps.

Potassium

The majority of dialysis centers use a fixed potassium dialysate which has been prepared centrally and delivered with a concentration of 01–02 mEq/L. Typically, one should not expect more than 80–100 mEq of potassium removal even with the use of a potassium free dialysate. The removal of excess potassium by dialysis is achieved by the use of a dialysate with a potassium concentration lower than that of plasma creating a gradient favoring potassium removal and its rate is largely a function of this gradient. Plasma potassium concentration falls rapidly in the early stages of dialysis, but as the plasma concentration falls, potassium removal becomes less efficient. Because potassium is freely permeable across the dialysis membrane, movement of potassium from the intracellular space to the extracellular space appears to be the limiting factor in potassium removal. Given the tendency for the plasma potassium to rise in the immediate postdialysis time period, the most efficient way to remove excess potassium stores would be to prescribe 2–3 hours periods of dialysis separated by several hours. The risk of arrhythmias is increased in the early stages of a dialysis session when the plasma potassium concentration may still be normal but rapidly declining. In patients who are at high risk for arrhythmias on dialysis, modeling the dialysate potassium concentration so as to maintain a constant blood to dialysate potassium gradient throughout the procedure may be of clinical benefit.

Bicarbonate

Bicarbonate is now the principal buffer used in dialysate. Producing bicarbonate dialysate requires a specifically designed system that mixes a bicarbonate concentrate and an acid concentrate with purified water. The acid concentrate contains a small amount of either lactic or acetic acid and all the calcium and magnesium. The exclusion of these cations from the bicarbonate concentrate prevents the precipitation of magnesium and calcium carbonate that would otherwise occur in the setting of a high bicarbonate concentration. During the mixing procedure the acid in the acid concentrate will react with an equimolar amount of bicarbonate to generate carbonic acid and carbon dioxide. The generation of carbon dioxide causes the pH of the final solution to fall to approximately 7.0–7.4. This more acidic pH as well as the lower concentrations of calcium and magnesium in the final mixture allow for these ions to remain in solution. The final concentration of bicarbonate in the dialysate is generally fixed in the range of 32–38 mmol/L. The bicarbonate level shown on the monitor of many dialysis machines that allow for adjusting dialysis solution bicarbonate by altering the concentrate proportioning ratio is the final bicarbonate concentration and does not take into account the acetate of sodium acetate that was produced from reaction of acetic acid with an equimolar amount of sodium bicarbonate which generates bicarbonate.

Dry Concentrates

Bicarbonate

In some machines, a cartridge containing dry sodium bicarbonate is used in place of a liquid "bicarbonate" concentrate. Use of dry bicarbonate cartridges obviates the problem of bacterial growth in "bicarbonate" concentrate and the concern of subsequent contamination of the final dialysis solutions.

Acid (Citric Acid or Sodium Diacetate)

While acetic acid is a liquid, dry "acid" concentrates can be made using either citric acid or sodium diacetate. The low concentration of citrate generated in citric acid-based dialysis solution may chelate plasma calcium that is adjacent to the dialysis membrane, impeding coagulation, improving dialyser clearance slightly, and increasing the dialyser reuse number. In dry acid concentrates containing citric acid (0.8 mM) plus a small amount (0.3 mM) of acetic acid, after mixing, the dialysis solution will contain 0.8 mM citrate (2.4 mEq/L) and 0.3 mM acetate, yielding about 2.7 mEq/L of bicarbonate-generating base.

Dialysate Magnesium

The usual concentration of magnesium in the dialysate is 0.5–1.0 mEq/L and is only rarely manipulated.

Dialysate Calcium

The dialysate calcium concentration is available as 1.25/1.5/1.75 mmol/L. The adjustment in the calcium is done depending on the clinical scenario and has implications with regard to metabolic bone disease, hemodynamic stability, and long-term effects on vascular calcification.

DIALYSATE PROPORTIONING SYSTEMS

These can be of three types:

1. **Type A:** Fixed volume of water, acid and bicarbonate concentrate.
2. **Type B:** Dynamic proportioning using conductivity measurement to control the acid and bicarbonate concentrate pumps.
3. **Type C:** Dynamic proportioning using a powder cartridge to prepare the bicarbonate concentrate online.

Several ratios of concentrate to water are available depending on the system, e.g., 01:1.225:32.775; 01:1.83:34; and 01:1.72:42.28. Some machines have fixed proportioning ratios while the newer ones have adjustable proportioning ratios.

Storing and Mixing Dialysis Concentrate

- The dialysis solution should be stored and dispensed as a drug.
- Educate all personnel about the type of dialysis solution in the unit. Ensure only authorize personnel handle the dialysis fluid. Do not dispense concentrates from large to small containers without a proper labeling system. Preferably containers for a single treatment should be kept in the unit.
- It is preferable to use only one bicarbonate concentrate system

SUGGESTED READING

1. Berube R. Sodium Bicarbonate Mixing Considerations. Horizons: A Supplement to Biomedical Instrumentation and Technology. 2006:59-65.
2. Desai N. Basics of base in hemodialysis solution: Dialysate buffer production, delivery and decontamination. Indian J Nephrol. 2015;25(4):189-93.
3. McGill RL, Weiner DE. Dialysate Composition for Hemodialysis: Changes and Changing Risk. Semin Dial. 2017;30(2):112-20.

Vascular Access: AV Fistula and Grafts

Kristin George, Shahbaj Ahmad, Hemant Mehta

INTRODUCTION

Vascular access is a critical aspect of delivering effective treatment to patients with end-stage renal disease (ESRD). It is the vascular access which allows the blood to be taken out from the patient's body into the dialysis machine (extracorporeal circuit) and return the filtered blood back to the patient.

A good vascular access should be:
- Easy to construct
- Provide adequate blood flow
- Have minimum complications
- Long lasting

Vascular access is the lifeline for end stage kidney disease (ESKD) patients. As a dialysis technician, one should have a sound understanding of the different types of vascular access, their management, and potential complications.

In this chapter we will try to understand various types of vascular access and its significance in hemodialysis.

There are three types of vascular access:
1. Arterio-venous fistula (AVF)
2. Arterio-venous graft (AVG)
3. Central venous catheter (CVC)

AVF was first described by Brescia and Cimino and remains the first choice for chronic hemodialysis patients. In this chapter we will discuss about AVF and AVG. The central venous catheter will be covered in the subsequent chapter.

AV FISTULA/AV GRAFT

An AV fistula is a surgically created connection between an artery and vein. This results in increased blood flow at high pressure through the vein, leading to enlargement and thickening of the venous segment. This is commonly done at the wrist between radial artery and cephalic vein. But can also be done at other sites like elbow and mid forearm.

An AV graft is also a connection of an artery and vein, but by a tube made of prosthetic material. The most commonly used material is polytetrafluoroethylene (PTFE) polymer.

The National Kidney Foundation's Kidney Disease Outcomes Quality Initiative (KDOQI) and the "Fistula First" initiative promote AV fistulas as the initial vascular access in at least 68% patients on dialysis.

Creation and Maturation Process

- During the AV fistula surgery, end on the vein is joined to the side of the artery to facilitate direct flow of blood from artery to vein.

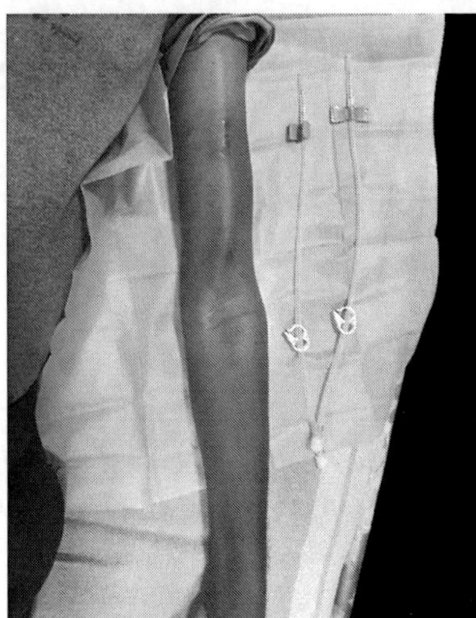

Fig. 1: Mature AV fistula with prominent straight venous segment. AVF cannulation needles are also seen in the picture.

- The fistula maturation process generally takes about 6–8 weeks and cannot be used immediately for dialysis.
- During the maturation process, the vein becomes dilated and the wall becomes thickened, which is the portion where the needles will be inserted for dialysis **(Fig. 1)**.
- It is important to monitor the fistula at each visit to assess for maturation and detect any signs of nonmaturation or delayed maturation for appropriate management.

Benefits and Advantages

Benefits AVF

- Lower rates of infection
- Higher patency rates
- Overall better patient survival

Benefits of AVG

- Can be used within 2 weeks of surgery
- Larger surface area for cannulation
- Easy cannulation

Disadvantages of AVF

- Cannot be used immediately
- Poor maturation rates in those with unsuitable vein or artery and elderly
- Pain related to needle prick/cannulation

Disadvantages of AVG

- Higher rates of stenosis and thrombosis
- Higher rates of infection compared to AVF (still less than catheters)

'Rule of 6' of Fistula Maturation

- 6 mm in diameter
- Less than 6 mm below the skin

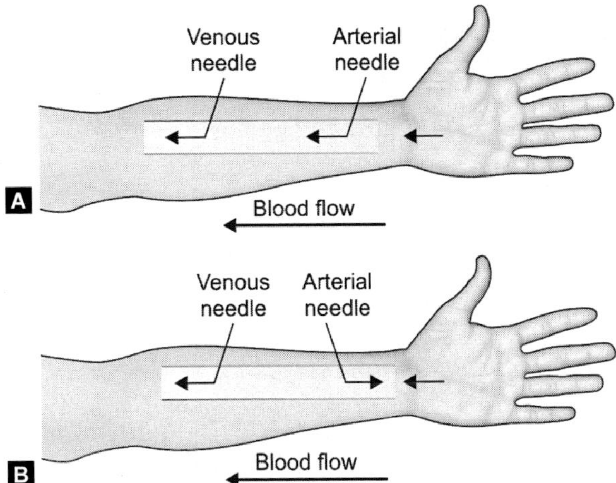

Figs. 2A and B: Direction of AVF needle insertion: (A) Both arterial and venous needle in the direction of venous return; (B) Arterial needle opposite to the direction of venous return. Note that the venous needle should always be in the direction of venous return.

- Blood flow of at least 600 mL/min
- 6 cm Straight segment for cannulation
- 6 Weeks maturation time

Any fistula should be allowed adequate time to mature before cannulating, as premature needle insertions can result in infiltration, hematoma and sometimes compression on the fistula resulting in permanent loss.

Cannulation of AVF/AVG

Two needles are inserted into the dilated segment of the vein. First the arterial needle is inserted and can be done either upstream or downstream direction. The venous needle is inserted in the direction of venous return **(Figs. 2A and B)**.

- **Step ladder technique:** The cannulation is done over a segment with each prick at a point slightly above the previous one, and this cycle continues **(Fig. 3)**.
- **Button hole/area cannulation technique:** The AVF is cannulated through the same site to create a tract. Once tract is formed, blunt needle is used to cannulate the fistula.

COMPLICATIONS

- **Stenosis:**
  - Narrowing of the AV fistula, commonly happens near the anastomotic site.
  - Can lead to poor flow and under-dialysis. Increases the risk of thrombosis.
- **Thrombosis:**
  - Blood clotting within the AV fistula can lead to AVF closure **(Fig. 4A)**.
  - It is the most common complication in AVF/AVG.
  - Causes include fistula compression, hematoma formation from cannulation injury, low blood pressure (BP), clotting abnormalities.
  - Antiplatelet drugs, early detection of stenosis and correction by elective angioplasty can help prevent thrombosis.
- **Infection:**
  - Redness, pain or pus discharge from the AVF/AVG

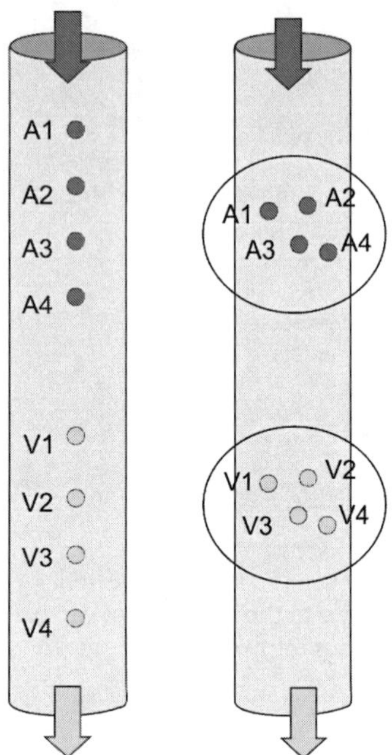

Fig. 3: Shows cannulation techniques of AVF.

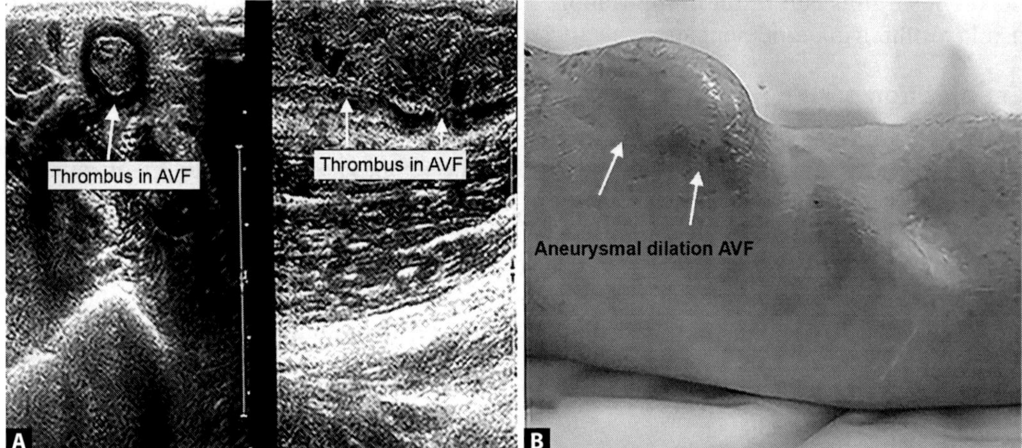

Figs. 4A and B: (A) Shows thrombus in AVF; (B) Shows aneurysmal dialtion of AVF.

- AV grafts can get infected more often than AV fistula
- Maintaining good hand hygiene practices can help in preventing infections

❖ **Hematoma formation:**

- Poor cannulation techniques or needle removal techniques can lead to extravasation and hematoma formation.
- If large can compress and result in thrombosis of the AVF.

❖ **Aneurysm:**

- Repeated cannulation in the same area can cause damage to the vessel wall resulting in dilatation and bulging **(Fig. 4B)**.
- Risk of rupture

- **Steal syndrome:**
  - Decreased blood supply to the distal arm due to retrograde flow of blood in the distal artery towards the AV fistula.
  - This can lead to symptoms of limb ischemia like pain, coldness, and abnormal sensations in the distal arm during dialysis.
  - If not corrected, can lead to ischemic ulcers and dry gangrene.

Meticulous handling of AV fistula and grafts, following appropriate steps of safe cannulation can go a long way in preventing complications and ensuring long life of the vascular access.

SUGGESTED READING

1. American Society of Diagnostic and Interventional Nephrology. http://www.asdin.org/.
2. https://www.cdc.gov/dialysis/: CDC Dialysis safety guidelines.
3. John TD, Peter GB, Todd SI. Handbook of Dialysis, 5th edition. Philadelphia, PA: Wolters Kluwer Health; 2014.
4. KDOQI. Clinical Practice Guideline for Vascular Access: 2019 Update. 2020;75(4):S1-164, SUPPLEMENT 2.

Vascular Access: Dialysis Catheters

10
CHAPTER

Kristin George, G Gireesh Reddy, Manas Ranjan Patel

INTRODUCTION

Hemodialysis catheter is a soft tube that is placed in a large vein, usually in the neck. It is estimated that more than 80% of the patients start dialysis on central venous catheter.

A hemodialysis catheter consists of two lumens—arterial and venous. The arterial lumen carries the blood away from the heart towards the dialysis machine and the venous lumen return the purified blood back to the patient's body.

Sites of Insertion

- Right and left internal jugular vein
- Femoral vein
- Subclavian vein
- **Others:** Translumbar IVC, external jugular vein, brachicephalic vein, etc.

The preferred site of insertion is the right internal jugular vein as it has a straight and short drainage pathway to the right atrium. The left internal jugular vein (IJV) catheter will have a longer and curved course of drain into the right heart **(Fig. 1)**.

TYPES

- Nontunneled (short-term and uncuffed)
- Tunneled catheter (long-term and cuffed)

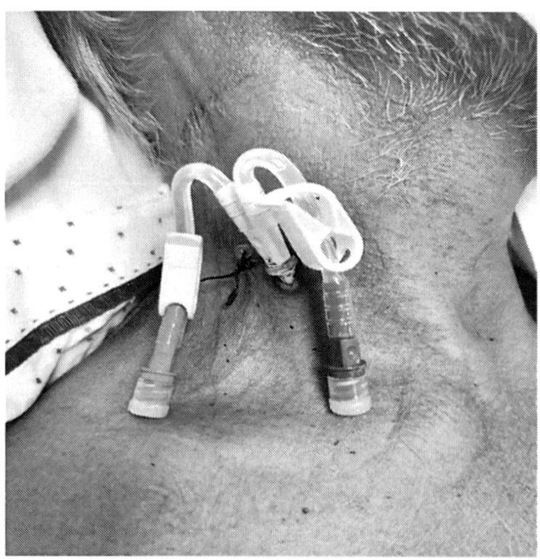

Fig. 1: Right IJV non tunneled catheter.

The nontunneled or short-term catheter has high risk of infections and prolonged use beyond 1–2 weeks should be avoided. Although in resource limited setting many a times, they are used for longer periods.

Tunneled catheter, also called 'Permcath' has a tunnel under the skin and a cuff near the exit site. The cuff is made up of Dacron and gets attached to the subcutaneous tissue in 4–6 weeks, thereby preventing entry of bacteria from the external surface. Whenever patient requires catheter beyond several weeks, cuffed catheters should be inserted to reduce the incidence of catheter-related infections **(Figs. 2 and 3)**.

Indications for Dialysis Catheters

- End stage kidney disease patient without mature AVF/AVG
- Patients on maintenance hemodialysis with dysfunction of AVF/AVG
- Acute renal failure
- Acute poisoning or overdose requiring hemodialysis
- Patients on CAPD (peritoneal dialysis) with peritonitis

Advantages of Catheters

- Can be used immediately after insertion
- Insertion can be done on OPD basis
- No need for inserting needles for dialysis

Disadvantages of Catheters

- Increased risk of infections
- Can cause stenosis of the central vein

Complications of Catheters

- **During insertion/immediate:**
  - Arterial puncture
  - Pneumothorax/hemothorax (accidental injury to lung)
  - Air embolism

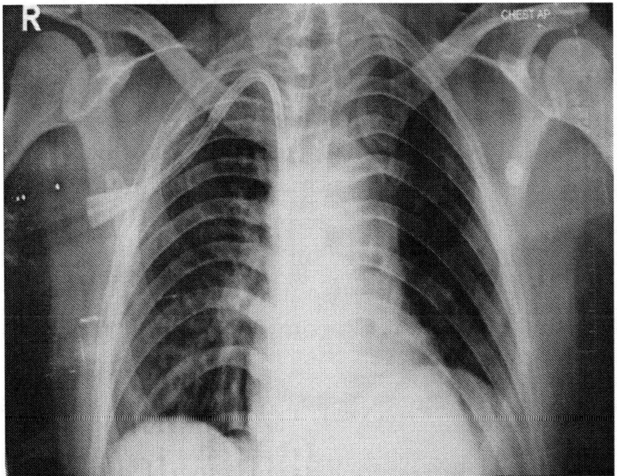

Fig. 2: Rt IJV catheter showing the straight course into right atrium.

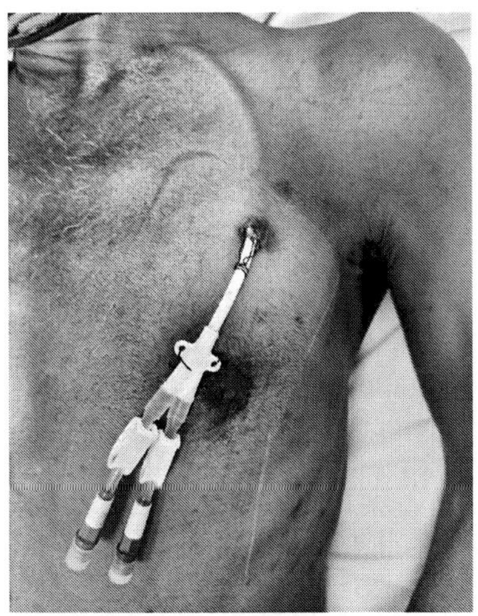

Fig. 3: Left IJV tunneled catheter.

- **Late complications:**
  - Thrombosis
  - Stenosis (more common with subclavian vein catheter)
  - Infection

Use of real-time ultrasound (USG) can significantly reduce the rate of complications during catheter insertion.

CATHETER CARE

Catheter-related blood stream infection (CRBSI) is an important cause for increased morbidity and mortality among patients on hemodialysis catheter. Following strict aseptic precautions and checklist of steps can help in reducing the rate of catheter infections:

- Under aseptic conditions, use clean gloves and mask while handling the catheter.
- After removal of dressing, examine the exit site for any redness/discharge.
- Wear sterile gloves and apply fresh dressing to the exit site.
- After cleaning the catheter ports, remove the caps and soak them in betadine or alcohol-based disinfectant.
- After aspirating the heparin lock solution from arterial and venous port, connect to the dialyser tubing.
- The exposure of the catheter hub to air should be minimized to prevent infections.
- After completion of dialysis, the catheter hubs should be soaked in antiseptic for 3–5 minutes. Chlorhexidine-based antiseptic solutions are found to be better than povidone iodine.
- Sterile dressing to be applied.

Bathing with Catheter In-situ

The exit site should not be immersed in water. Direct pouring of water over the catheter is to be avoided. In case of tunnelled catheters, once the exit tunnel is healed, showering can be permitted, preferably before coming for dialysis, so that fresh dressing can be applied.

Catheter Locks

- **Heparin:** After completion of dialysis, the catheter ports are filled with heparin at a concentration of about 1,000–5,000 U/mL. This is to prevent clot formation within the lumen. The volume of heparin to be instilled depends on the length of the arterial and venous ports and is usually labeled on the catheter hub.
- **Citrate 4%:** It can be used in place of heparin to prevent blood clotting. Some studies have shown citrate to be better than heparin in preventing infections in the catheter. But as citrate chelates calcium, there is an increased risk of hypocalcemia and arrhythmia if higher concentration or quantity is injected.
- **Other locks:** EDTA, ethanol containing catheter locks have been used in an attempt to reduce the rate of infections. Antibiotic lock solutions are also used in specific situations but universal use in all patients to prevent infections is not recommended as it can lead to increased drug resistance.
- **Exit site ointment:** Mupirocin ointment at the catheter exit site can be used till healing or in patients with repeated infections.
- **Nasal decolonization:** Use of intranasal mupirocin to remove staphylococcus colonization prior to catheter insertion has been shown to be effective in reducing the rate of infections.

Catheter Infections

CRBSI is the leading cause of catheter dysfunction, catheter loss, patient morbidity and mortality among patients. Most of the infections arise from contamination of the catheter ports by dialysis surface or hands of healthcare professionals. It can also be from the skin flora of the patient.

- **Exit site infections:** Erythema, tenderness, pus discharge from the exit site, without any tenderness over the tunnel. It can be treated with local antibiotic cream.
- **Tunnel infection:** Tenderness and swelling along the tunnel. May need catheter removal.
- **Catheter-related blood stream infection (CRBSI):** Patients have fever, chills, hypotension, which worsen during dialysis.
  - Paired blood culture should be sent from the catheter and peripheral line.
  - Empirical antibiotics should be started covering both gram positive (e.g., vancomycin) and gram negative (e.g., amikacin) organisms.
  - Antibiotic locks may be used along with systemic therapy.

SUGGESTED READING

1. Clinical Practice Guidelines for the Diagnosis and Management of Intravascular Catheter-Related Infection: 2009. Update by the Infectious Diseases Society of America.
2. Diagnosis, prevention and treatment of hemodialysis catheter-related bloodstream infections (CRBSI): a position statement of European Renal Best Practice (ERBP).
3. https://www.cdc.gov/dialysis/: CDC Dialysis safety guidelines.
4. John TD, Peter GB, Todd SI. Handbook of Dialysis, 5th edition. Philadelphia, PA: Wolters Kluwer Health; 2014.
5. KDOQI. Clinical Practice Guideline for Vascular Access: 2019 Update.2020;75(4):S1-164, SUPPLEMENT 2.

Dialysis: Initiation and Termination

11
CHAPTER

Debashish Mahapatra, Ayan Dey, Umesh Khanna

INTRODUCTION

Hemodialysis (HD) sessions no matter how mundane and routine they seem, is nevertheless stressful, especially the first one. And this stress is beyond a physical one. Every dialysis technician needs to remember this while attending to a patient, as often they are the interface between a patient and the nephrologist/doctor.

INITIATION

This section will deal with the activities one needs to do while initiating a particular HD session for a patient [either maintenance HD or HD in acute kidney injury (AKI)]. For ease of understanding, we have divided these activities to—1. Patient-related and 2. Therapy-related.

Patient-related

- Greet the patient with a smile and address him/her with respect acceptable for the place or region (like 'How are you Mr Saini' or 'Namashkaram Mr Damodaran'). Check how they have been doing since the last HD session, while stressing on any problem related to last HD session like fever, pain at the access site.
- Check about meal (prior light meal is desirable) and medications, particularly anti-hypertensives, and antidiabetic medications.
- Check 'HD prescription' if any, given by doctor/nephrologist; especially important for patients of AKI, anticoagulation type and dose, any medication to be given like iron or antibiotic, erythropoiesis stimulating agent dose, etc.
- Check vital parameters and body weight. Inform HD center in-charge if anything is grossly abnormal (e.g., blood pressure high or particularly low, body weight gains higher than usual).

New Patient

- Check the need for HD and prescription (particularly important for a patient of end stage renal disease, as the initial few sessions are truncated to avoid 'dialysis disequilibrium syndrome').
- Check lab reports (particularly HBs Ag, anti-HCV and anti-HIV status, as many centers practice segregation).
- Check the availability of dialysis access.
- Counseling and consent are extremely important and should be done deliberately and diligently, to avoid any chances of miscommunication. A specimen of the 'Consent form' is attached as **Appendix A.** Separate counseling and consent should be obtained for HD access creation.

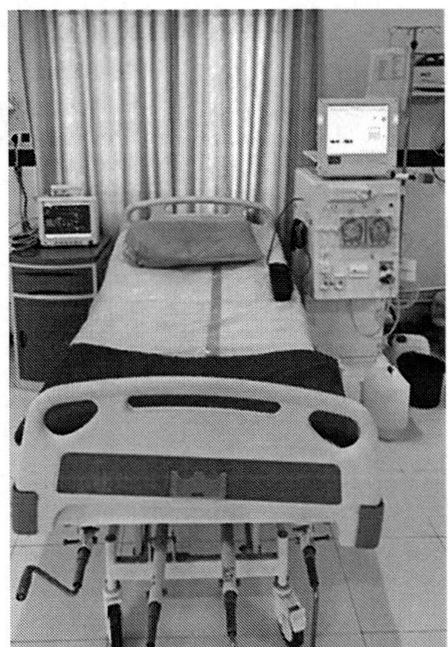

Fig. 1: A bed ready to receive patient.

- Keep the bed ready beforehand with a fresh bedsheet, pillow cover and blanket **(Fig. 1)**. Priming fluid, fistula needles should be kept ready by the bedside.
- Make the patient to lie or recline on the bed comfortably.

Therapy-related

- Ideally 2–3 dialysis technicians are required to attend to the patient when HD is being started. While one fetches the dialyser and makes the machine ready, the other inspects and readies the access.
- Inspect access, check for redness/discharge from the exit site and flow after withdrawing the heparin lock from temporary access. If the patient is having arteriovenous fistula (AVF) then check for redness, skin breaks and thrill.
- Clean with antiseptic solution and prepare AVF for canulation. Arterial-side needle should be directed towards the fistula and venous-side needle away from it and both separated by at least 5 cm to avoid recirculation **(Fig. 2)**. In case of temporary access/catheter, after antiseptic application open hub and withdraw first to remove heparin or locking solution **(Fig. 3)**. Predialysis blood sampling may be done at this point.
- Acid or Part 'A' and base or Part 'B' is available as powder concentrates and needs to be prepared in a mixer with recommended volume of water. Part 'A' is also commercially available as premixed solution. If both are being prepared in same mixer, then thorough cleaning is required to avoid intermixing.

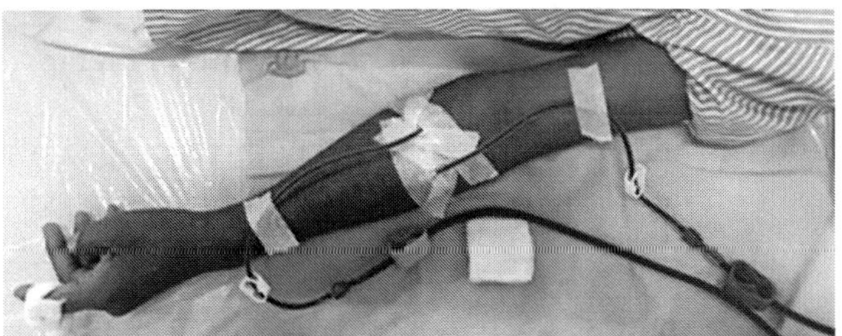

Fig. 2: Arteriovenous fistula access with attached AVF needles and HD tubing. Note that arterial-side needle is pointing towards the fistula anastomosis and venous-side needle away from it.

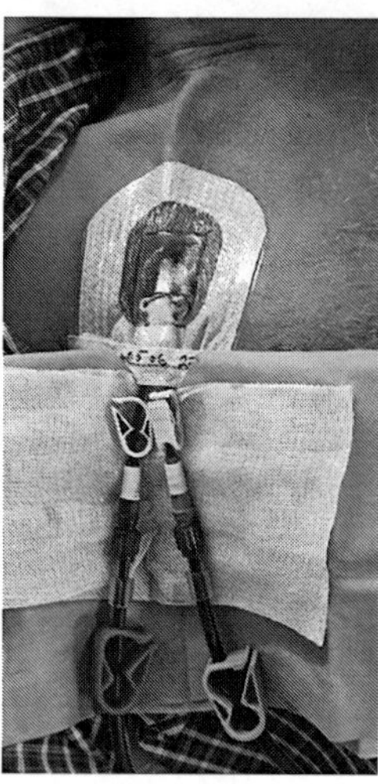

Fig. 3: A tunnelled and cuffed HD catheter in internal jugular vein on the right side with attached HD tubing. Note red to red and blue to the blue attachment.

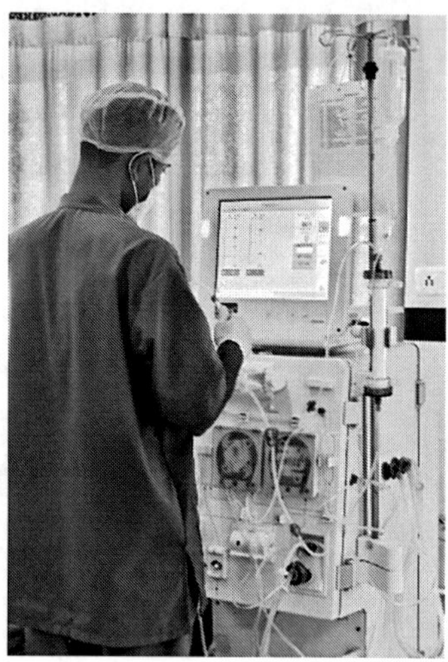

Fig. 4: Priming being undertaken on a B Braun Dialog + machine with dialyser and tubing already connected. Note that dialyser couplings and concentrate line couplings are attached with the machine at this point. *(For color version, see Plate 5)*

- Part 'A' and Part 'B' solutions are kept ready. Retrieve dialyser and tubing if being reused and flush with normal saline as per center protocol. Inspect dialyser for cracks to any part. Reuse of dialyser requires greater flush volume to wash-off blood and disinfectant. A new dialyser requires half to 1 liter normal saline (NS) flush and reuse requires 2–3 liters. Attach dialyser and tubing to machine and fill with heparinized saline **(Fig. 4)**.
- Set machine to HD mode and connect arterial-side-port first and let blood come up till the venous-side-port. This process discards the extra heparinized saline from dialyser and tubing. Then connect venous-side-port to patient. Set anticoagulation mode to run, like heparin infusion/timed boluses or regional heparin or citrate anticoagulation.
- Set dialysis time, blood flow and dialysate flow rate, ultrafiltration (UF) volume and conductivity. UF volume is calculated as UF = weigh gain (i.e., present weight of patient – Dry weight) + any requisite volume to be infused in form of blood, therapy, or injection. Conductivity is usually not changed unless any electrolyte abnormality is existing.
- During therapy watch for alarms, vital parameters, and any difficulty to patient.

TERMINATION

Termination is usually done at end of therapy time or earlier in case of complications. Like during initiation, 2–3 technicians are required for termination too.

- Anticoagulation should be stopped in last half to one hour of therapy. Check machine and patient parameters at end of therapy.
- Return blood to patient by flushing with NS. Blood pump is used for the same.
- Inspect access site and remove tubing attachments from access. If temporary or catheter access is there, then clean access site and hub with antiseptic solution, apply locking solution or heparin, close hub and do dressing of site. In case of AVF, remove one needle at a time and apply pressure for 5–10 min check for clotting or no bleeding at puncture site, apply antiseptic and do a pressure bandage. Always check for thrill in AVF at this point. Blood sampling may be done after a preset time after termination and before closure of access.

- Patient can now be removed from bed and body-weight taken. He/she should be asked to be in waiting room for sometime before heading home as an extra precaution. Parameters like pre- and post-HD bodyweight and blood pressure, UF volume, therapy time, any injection or medication given, and complications should be documented.
- Remove Part 'A' and Part 'B' concentrate lines are removed and rinsed as per manufacturer specifications. Dialyser and tubing are removed and processed if reuse is intended. Label dialyser with full name of patient, number of reuse and date of last use before storing. If reuse is not intended, then break either blood or dialysate hubs of the dialyser and cut the tubing before discarding in appropriate-color waste bags, to prevent misuse.
- HD machine should be brought to a short disinfection mode before next therapy and surface of machine thoroughly wiped with an antiseptic solution, taking special care of knobs and hubs. All spare needles and syringes are discarded.

SUGGESTED READING

1. Chan CT, Blankestijn PJ, Dember LM, Gallieni M, Harris DCH, Lok CE, Mehrotra R, Stevens PE, Wang AY, Cheung M, Wheeler DC, Winkelmayer WC, Pollock CA; Conference Participants. Dialysis initiation, modality choice, access, and prescription: Conclusions from a Kidney Disease: Improving Global Outcomes (KDIGO). Kidney Int. 2019;96(1):37-47.
2. Standard Of Care For Maintainance Hemodialysis In India. Ministry of Health & Family Welfare Govt. of India. 2010.

Maintenance of Dialysis Machine and Bicarbonate Mixer

12
CHAPTER

Debashish Mahapatra, Dharmendra S Bhadauria, Narayan Prasad

INTRODUCTION

Maintenance of dialysis machines is a vital part of the functioning of the dialysis center and needs to be undertaken with diligence. Center maintenance protocol should be rigid with no scope for amiss. Primarily, maintenance activities are directed towards limiting downtime of machines, but will also achieve confidence build-up among patients, and dialysis technicians alike. It also has bearing on dialysis dose delivery.

The frequency of maintenance activity can be:

- Per treatment
- Daily or alternate days
- Weekly
- Monthly
- Quarterly
- Semi-annually and annually
- Per machine running hours

A different set of maintenance activities may be defined as per periodicity. In this chapter, we will limit ourselves to the maintenance of dialysis machines and bicarbonate mixers.

MAINTENANCE OF DIALYSIS MACHINE

Disinfection

Disinfection done properly protects against outbreaks of hepatitis B and C and other bacterial sepsis in the center. In this regard, disinfection may be considered in two parts—external and internal disinfection.

1. **External disinfection:** External disinfection or surface cleaning should mandatorily be done after each treatment session and is a broad term that includes not only disinfection of HD machine surfaces but also of other surfaces which have come in contact with patients like blood pressure measuring cuffs, dialysis bed, etc. Special attention should be paid to cleaning if there have been any blood spills. Special attention should be given to the parts of HD machines where the dialyser and acid/base concentrate couplings are attached, as sediments tend to settle there. The touch screen should be in 'off' mode for wiping or cleaning. The suggested 'Check list' is attached as **Appendix B**.

   Alcohol-based solutions are ideal because of their low cost, ease of availability, and effect on a variety of organisms; they are also mild on the skin and eye, and inhalation does not cause irritation. Ethyl or isopropyl alcohol (not more than 70% solution) can be used for this purpose and are widely bactericidal, fungicidal, and viricidal with limited effect on spores. 1% Sodium hypochlorite or bleach can also be used and is effective on bacteria, fungi, and viruses, but the effect on spores is limited at this concentration. This should not be used on touch screens and can cause irritation to the skin and eye on exposure.

2. **Internal disinfection and decalcification:** Internal disinfection is required to remove any microorganism contamination and biofilm. Internal disinfection frequency is a matter of debate and should be adjusted to utility vs convenience. All relevant guidelines recommend external disinfection after each treatment, irrespective of the patient's blood-borne virus infection status. Internal disinfection is not recommended between patients, even when a blood leak is suspected, though center practices may vary. As most newer HD machines are 'Single Pass' type and there is no recirculation of outflowing dialysate disinfection with a manufacturer-recommended disinfectant after a day's treatments are over, is adequate. However, most manufacturers recommend the use of decalcifying disinfectant (citric acid 50%) between treatments to regularly remove deposits of calcium and magnesium bicarbonate from the internal circuitry.

When using any disinfectant other than citric acid 50%, testing for residual disinfectant presence is necessary and if presence is detected then further rinsing should be done till residual disinfectant testing is negative. If bleach is used for disinfection, then thermal disinfection should follow to remove residual bleach.

The process of disinfection is automated and an example of available options in a B Braun **(Fig. 1)** Dialog + machine is given in **Figures 1 to 4.** The suggested steps for internal disinfection are given in **Appendix C.**

Maintenance

Maintenance may be classified into in-center and preventive maintenance. Preventive maintenance is carried out by trained personnel at manufacturer-recommended intervals and should be strictly followed. The preventive maintenance includes the replacement of any wear and tear parts aimed at the fault-free operation of the HD machine and details of such activity are beyond the scope of this book.

In-center maintenance should include the following:

- Daily inspection of the machine for leakage, rusting, sediment deposit.
- Disinfection as discussed earlier.
- Regular change of Diasafe or Diacap filter, as specified interval recommended by the manufacturer.

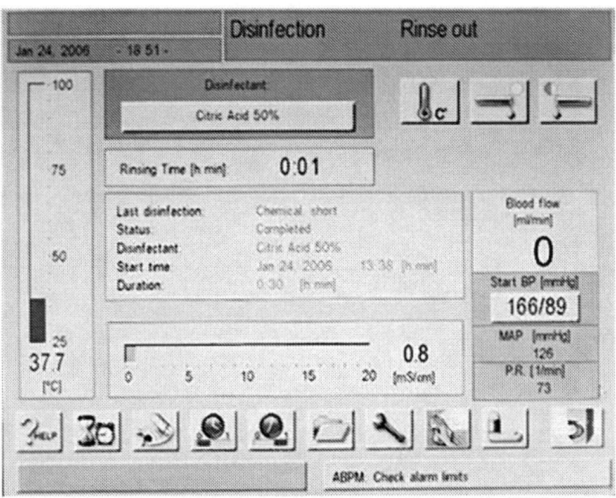

Fig. 1: Disinfection options in a B Braun Dialog + HD machine. Note options of thermal, full and short chemical disinfections. If none of the options are selected, then the machine remains in 'Rinse Mode' and during this internal circuits are rinsed or washed with ultrapure water. *(For color version, see Plate 6)*

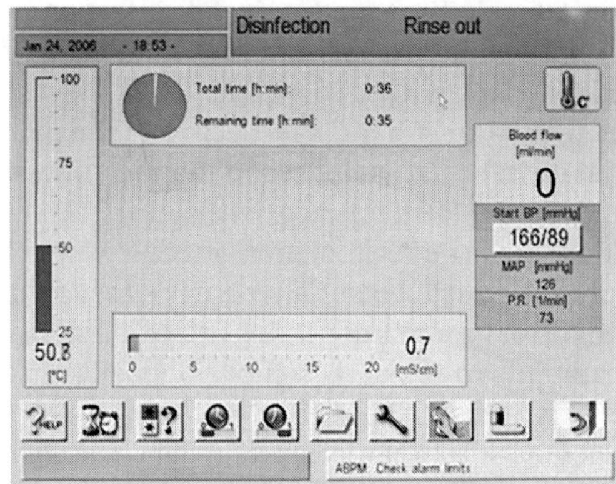

Fig. 2: Thermal disinfection has been selected.
Note the total time of 36 minutes is required for this.

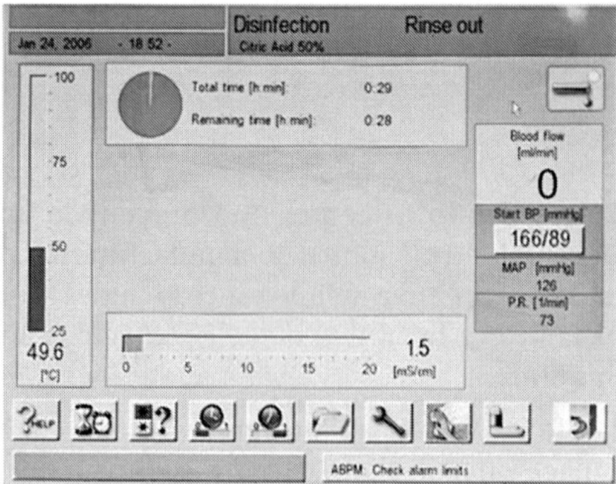

Fig. 3: Full chemical disinfection with citric acid 50% has been selected.
Note the total time required is 29 minutes for this. Time for disinfection will change with the change of disinfectant.

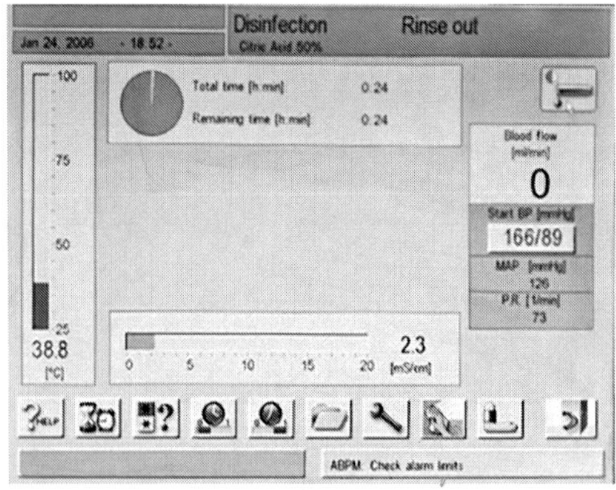

Fig. 4: Short chemical disinfection with citric acid 50% has been selected.
Note the total time required is 24 minutes for this. Time for disinfection will change with the change of disinfectant.

BICARBONATE MIXER

Bicarbonate concentrate mixers are available from a wide variety of manufacturers and are an assembly of a motor and a drum made of medical-grade plastic or stainless steel, with an agitator and micro-processor-controlled proportioning system, in which volume control, mixing, and dispensation are automated. At times the same mixer can be used for both bicarbonate and acid concentrates but should be thoroughly rinsed in between the two processes. Some dialysis units even use semi-automatic washing machines for this purpose!

After mixing the bicarbonate concentrate may be delivered to the HD machine through a delivery loop or simply in containers. Some HD machines use prefilled cartridges or bags containing sodium bicarbonate attached directly and when mixed with RO water allow the creation of base concentrate at the point of use. Bicart (Gambro) and Bibag (Fresenius) are two such cartridges that are widely used.

When a bicarbonate mixer is used and delivery of concentrate is through a closed loop or in containers, the whole arrangement needs disinfection, as bicarbonate provides an excellent medium for bacterial growth and biofilm formation, and periodic removal of carbonate deposits and should include the loop-delivery system and containers as applicable.

Disinfection may be carried out with sodium hypochlorite (bleach) or a commercially available cleansing solution containing acetic or peracetic acid. Additional cleaning to remove carbonate deposits is required when using bleach for disinfection, but not when using commercially available cleansing solutions containing acetic or peracetic acid. The suggested steps of disinfection are given in **Appendix D**.

SUGGESTED READING

1. Ahmad TA. The Influence of Maintenance Quality of Hemodialysis Machines on Hemodialysis Efficiency. Saudi J Kidney Dis Transplant. 2009;20(1):49-56.
2. Desai N. Basics of base in hemodialysis solution: Dialysate buffer production, delivery and decontamination. Indian J Nephrol. 2015;25(4):189-93.
3. Dialysis Station Routine Disinfection. Centers for Disease Control and Prevention National Center for Emerging and Zoonotic Infectious Diseases. www.cdc.gov/dialysis checklist.
4. KDIGO 2022 Clinical Practice Guideline for the Prevention, Diagnosis, Evaluation, and Treatment of Hepatitis C in Chronic Kidney Disease. Kidney Int. 2022;102(6S):S129-205.
5. Reimer R. Hemodialysis machine disinfection: A safe period of time between cycles. CANNT J. 2000;10(2):23-5.
6. Stragier A, Jadoul M. Should dialysis machines be disinfected between patients' shifts? EDTNA ERCA J. 2003;29(2):73-6.

RO Water and Water Treatment Plant

13
CHAPTER

Ramanjit Singh Akal, Nikhil Bhasin, J Balasubramaniam

INTRODUCTION

In the normal dialysis treatment, approximately 120–200 liters of water is used. The quality of water is utmost important as the contaminants in the water can accumulate several folds in the body of patients in presence of renal failure. Hence the chemical as well as microbiological purity of the water is required which is supplied from municipality which already contains chlorine or chloramine which poses several health-related issues like hemolysis in a renal failure patient. There are other impurities **(Table 1)** which causes significant effects like aluminum (adynamic bone disease and dialysis encephalopathy syndrome), fluoride (ventricular fibrillations), chlorine, chloramine, copper and zinc (hemolytic anemia). There are bacteria and bacterial toxins causing fever and untoward reactions affecting patient condition. These all impurities are required to be purified as per Association for Advancement of Medical Instrumentation (AAMI) standards before using this water for dialysis at dialysis facility **(Table 2)**.

Table 1: Water contaminant acceptable levels.

Contaminant	*Suggested maximum allowable levels (mg/mL)*
Calcium	2
Magnesium	4
Sodium	70
Potassium	8
Fluoride	0.2
Chloride	0.5
Chloramines	0.1
Nitrates	2.0
Sulfate	100
Copper, barium and zinc	Each 0.1
Aluminum	0.01
Arsenic, lead and silver	Each 0.005
Cadmium	0.001
Chromium	0.114
Selenium	0.09
Mercury	0.0002

Table 2: AAMI microbiological standards for dialysis water.			
Microbiological level	*Maximum allowable level*	*Action level*	*Ultrapure dialysate*
Colony forming unit (CFU)	<100 CFU/mL	>50 CFU/mL	<0.1 CFU/mL
Endotoxin level	<0.25 EU/mL	>0.125 EU/mL	<0.03 EU/mL

WATER TREATMENT PLANT (FIG. 1)

Various steps in purification process:

1. **Temperature blending valve:** It keeps the temperature of the feed water constant to keep the efficiency of reverse osmosis (RO) membrane optimum.
2. **Acid feed systems:** It keeps the source water pH between 7 and 8 by adding hydrochloric acid if it's alkaline. The excessive alkalinity reduces efficiency of carbon beds.
3. **Raw water tank:** This is storage of source water in a big tank.
4. **Booster pumps:** It required to maintain the velocity and pressure of the water constant in the closed system.
5. **Multimedia filter:** It's the first filter in the pathway of source water resulting in settling of particulate matter less then 10 microns by sedimentation. This is made up from multiple layers of gravel, sand, and anthracite. Any malfunction at this level, can result in damage to RO membrane. To prevent its clogging, daily backwashing is required to be conducted after the dialysis treatment. The pressure gauges are to be present, both pre and postmultimedia filter to document any change in pressure. The pressure changes greater then 10 mm Hg indicates its malfunction.

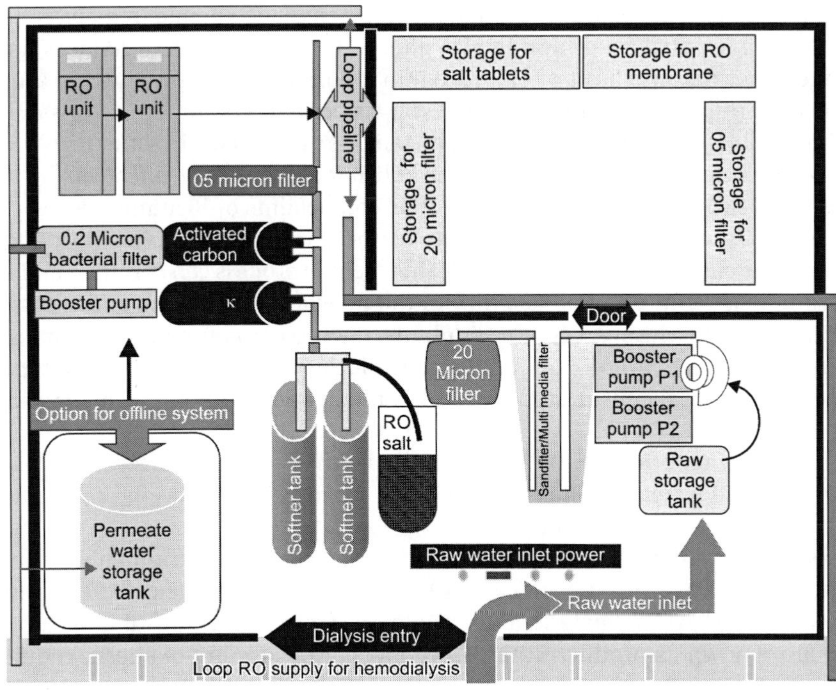

Fig. 1: Schematic diagram of water treatment plant of standard hemodialysis center.

6. **Water softener:** This is meant to reduce the hardness of the source water, which occurs due to retention of divalent calcium and magnesium salts resulting in malfunction of RO membrane due to scaling. The process of softening occurs due to presence of ion exchange resin, which exchange sodium ions in place of calcium and magnesium ions present in hard water. The brine tank contains supersaturated sodium chloride solution which help in regeneration of resin (releases sodium ion) for exchange with calcium and magnesium ions. The hardness of water is measured in parts per million (PPM) or grains per gallon (GPG). The water hardness is checked with colorimetric test strips preferably at the end of the day. Once treated the hardness should be less then 17 PPM or 1 GPG. The brine tank is also required to be checked regularly for sufficiency of sodium chloride pellets which are required to be above the level of water.
7. **Ultra-filters:** These are extra filters which are placed in the circuit of water treatment to separate remaining particulate matter which escaped the filtration process. These are placed after multimedia filter and after carbon filter to catch particulate matter and bacteria as well as endotoxin escaping previous filters. Their size may vary from 0.001 to 20 microns. These are required to be exchanged timely as they get clogged with debris and results in pressure drop across the filter. The pressure drop is required to be checked daily and the filter is required be changed id drop in pressure is significant. The regular monitoring of pressure drop across the water softener is required to be carried out and any drop of pressure greater then 10 mm Hg indicates malfunction of resin bed. The softener regeneration must occur once the dialysis hours are complete and there must be check for the conductivity by conductivity monitors, raising alarm if the concentration of sodium exceeds certain fixed limit.
8. **Carbon tanks:** With the use of activated carbon, chlorine and chloramine are removed from the water, which are added by municipal corporations to prevent bacterial growth. The inadequate removal may present as severe hemolytic anemia in dialysis dependent patients. The residual free chlorine also affects RO membrane and reduces its life. The maximum permissible limit of chlorine and chloramine in treated water are 0.5 PPM and 01 PPM respectively. The chlorine testing is done by colorimetric strips or by online monitoring. In this process, the two carbon tanks are connected in series in which the first one is worker carbon and the other one is polisher carbon. To be effective, the minimum contact time of 5 minutes in each tank or total contact time of 10 minutes is to be ensured. The chlorine sample is to be taken for assessment from the sampling port after worker carbon. If the chlorine level is acceptable, the dialysis process can continue and if it is not, then sample is required to be taken from the polisher carbon tank and assessed. If the chlorine levels are within acceptable limits, the dialysis can continue(with remedial action required for worker carbon tank), but if the chlorine levels are more the acceptable, the dialysis is to immediately be stopped, with remedial action for both worker and polisher carbon.
9. **Empty bed contact time (EBCT):** This is the method to estimate contact time between carbon bed and water. It represents EBCT = V/Q where V denotes the carbon volume in the tank and Q denotes the flow rate.
10. **Reverse osmosis (RO) plant:** In this process, water is pushed through tight membrane with the help of pressure which causes blockade to the passage of different impurities like particulate matter, bacteria and endotoxins (*refer* **Tables 1 and 2**) as a result pure water also known as product water is produced. The amount of energy required to do this process depends upon source water conductivity. The RO system consists of number of filters, membrane, pumps, and various monitors, through which source water is put

and product water is formed. The efficiency of RO system depends upon the quality and temperature of source water. Most of the water treatment systems have 02 ROs connected for better function, but it's not mandatory if the quality of source water is good. For optimal functioning, the pressure, flowrate, and conductivity of the water are required to be checked regularly.

Water Distribution Loop (Online System)

This loop is made up of polyvinyl chloride (PVC) or cross-linked polyethylene (PEX) piping's (compatible with heat sterilization) which are smooth, don't have any gaps or ridges and have minimum joints which prevents any stagnancy and hence prevents growth of bacteria or biofilm formation.

SUGGESTED READING

1. Dheda S, Van Eps C, Hawley C, Johnson DW. Water Treatment for Centre and Home-Based Hemodialysis [Internet]. Updates in Hemodialysis. InTech; 2015. Available from: http://dx.doi.org/10.5772/59380.
2. John TD, Peter GB, Todd SI. Handbook of Dialysis, 5th edition. Philadelphia, PA: Wolters Kluwer Health; 2014.
3. Nissenson AR. Handbook of dialysis therapy, 1st south Asia edition.

Dialyser Reprocessing

Ramanjit Singh Akal, Vineet Behera, SR Gedela

INTRODUCTION

It is the set of process in which dialyser is treated as per association for the advancement of medical instrumentation (AAMI) standards, so that it can be used multiple times. The processes make it safe as well as effective for use, but as the cost of dialysers have reduced, the reprocessing of dialyser being followed to reduce the financial burden on patients as well as to reduce the environmental waste generation.

Do's and Don'ts for Dialyser Reprocessing

- The reprocessing unit must have adequate reprocessing standard operating procedure (SOP) protocol.
- Adequate personal protective devices to be worn during the reprocessing to limit the risk of infection.
- There should be adequate system for checking the adequacy of reprocessing by performance testing and not only visual inspection of dialysers.
- The performance test results are to be checked and documented by operator staff as well as the decision to discard the dialyser is to be taken by operator staff.
- Only the dialyser approved by manufacturer for reuse may be reprocessed.
- HIV and HBV positive patient's dialysers should not be reprocessed.
- Processing of HCV positive patients to be done in designated reprocessing area.
- The dialyser headers, end caps, O rings and tubing may be reprocessed along with dialyser but arterial as well as venous transducer protectors to be avoided.
- Chemical reprocessing is preferred in general, except in case of polysulfone dialysers in which heat reprocessing is to be done.
- The use of automated reprocessing machine is recommended if available.
- Daily disinfection of reprocessing machine is to be done with sodium hypochlorite as well as weekly calibration of the reprocessing machine to be carried out with sodium hypochlorite.

REPROCESSING METHODS

There are two methods of reprocessing as mentioned:

1. **Manual method:** The various steps of reprocessing process is done manually by the operator. **(Figs. 1A to F)**.
2. **Automated method:** In this method, the various steps of reprocessing are done by automated machine, which makes it more consistent and avoid human slip-ups **(Fig. 2)**.

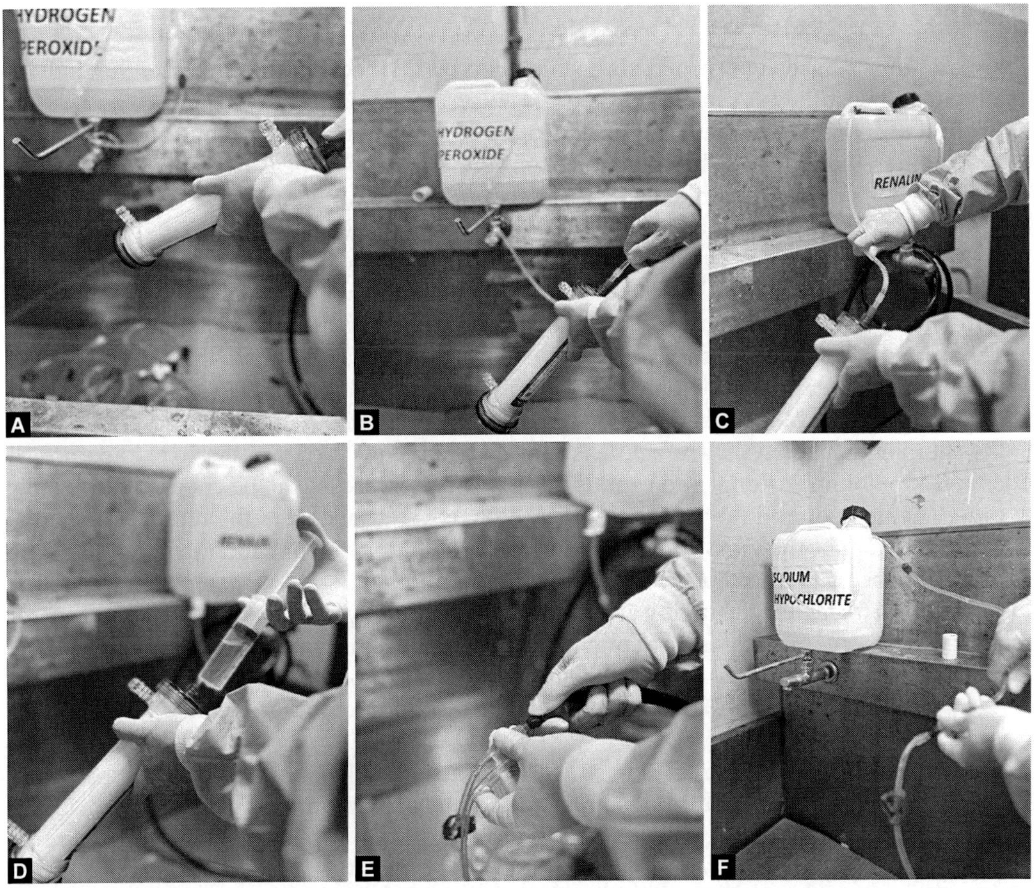

Figs. 1A to F: (A) Manual washing: Flushing of dialyser with RO water; (B) Filling of hydrogen peroxide in dialyser; (C) Measuring total cell volume using 50 mL syringe; (D) Filling of renalin; (E) AV tubing flushing with RO water; (F) Filling of sodium hypochlorite solution in AV tubing. *(For color version, see Plate 7)*

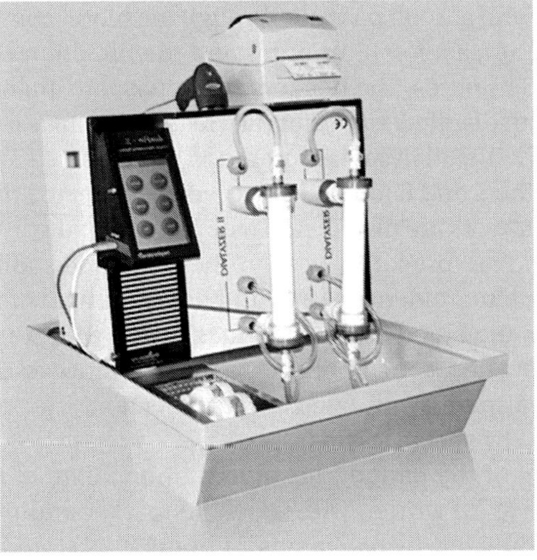

Fig. 2: Automated dialyser reprocessing system.

PHASES OF REPROCESSING

There are three phases of reprocessing which can be divided into prefirst use, the dialysis treatment and postdialysis phase.

1. **Prefirst use:** In this the, new dialyser is allotted to the patient and his name and his patient ID is written indelibly. His baseline total cell volume (TCV) is measured and pressure leak is checked. It is rinsed and filled with disinfectant.
2. **The dialysis treatment:** The dialyser is inspected for clotted fibers. The presence of disinfectant is confirmed by inspection (both headers have to be 2/3 filled) and by test strips. Adequate contact time of the disinfectant is to be confirmed. The dialyser is primed with normal saline for 15–30 minutes. The trapped air is removed by timely rotating the dialyser. The strip test is repeated to confirm, no residual disinfectant activity in dialysis circuit. Before instituting the treatment the dialysis prescription is confirmed.
3. **Postdialysis:** The blood is returned to the patient with the help of heparinized saline after the completion of dialysis. The saline is allowed to circulate for 5 minutes in extracorporeal circuit after joining arterial and venous tubing. The pressure leak to be checked during this time. The dialyser and tubing are transported in covered bucket to the reprocessing area, in order to reduce the cross contamination to the operator staff or with other dialysers. The procedure being followed postdialysis is under mentioned.
    - *Rinsing with water:* The tubing are removed from the dialyser and it's blood compartment and dialyser compartment are connected to the water (minimum AAMI standard) source. The pressure gradient is to be created from dialysate to blood compartment for 30 minutes till clear effluent comes out. The headers are also required to be cleaned for deposited lipids and clots.
    - *1% Hypochlorite instillation:* The 1% hypochlorite is instilled into the blood compartment for contact time of <2 minutes and immediately rinse out. If hydrogen peroxide or renalin (peracetic acid-based reagent) is used, then it must be in dialysate compartment and reverse ultrafiltration or backwashing to be done after 2 minutes of exposure. The backwashing or reverse ultrafiltration is done by connecting the one end of blood compartment to the waters supply and keeping the other end open. The one end of dialysate compartment is connected to water source through Hansen's connector and the other dialysate end is capped. The water is pushed through dialysate compartment at the pressure 1.3 bar and should pass out through the blood compartment. The procedure is to be carried out at least for 15 minutes and the direction of the flow to be reversed alternatively every 5 minutes. The headers are removable, than these along with O rings are to be cleaned with disinfectant. Later the cleaning agent is to be rinsed out with water.
    - *Inspection of dialyser:* The dialyser is required to be inspected for obvious clots in header, change in color of fibers and if found more than 20% affected then dialyser is discarded.
    - *Disinfection:* The dialysers are disinfected with freshly made disinfectants which are kept in 50 liters tanks and are prepared weekly. These include sodium hypochlorite (1–2%), formaldehyde (4%), glutaraldehyde (2%) and peracetic acid or renalin (3.5%). In view of accumulation of air, the blood compartment is rinsed with water, so that air is removed and disinfectant is pushed from other side so that it removes water. It is recommended to have both the compartments fully filled with disinfectant. The presence of the disinfectant activity is confirmed by specific strip tests.
    - *Labeling:* The name of the patient, hospital number, date of reprocessing, number of reuses and TCV are to be written with indelible marker and pasted to the dialyser. The minimum contact time for disinfectant is 24 hours. It is stored in sealed bag in specific rack for the patient. It is required to be reprocessed if not used within 7 days.

- *Reprocessing of tubing:* The tubing is also treated similarly. These are first washed with RO water to clean any blood, followed by 1.6%
- *Test of performance:* The methods of checking the performance includes pressure leak test and total cell volume (TCV) or fiber bundle volume (FBV).
  - Pressure leak test: It is to be done at during priming. The saline is filled in venous bubble trap till it is 2/3 filled. The venous pressure transducer is connected to it. The blood pump is started at 100–150 mL/min with venous outflow clamped. Once the venous pressure increases up to 400 mm Hg, the blood pump is stopped and the rate fall of pressure is observed. If fall is more than 1 mm Hg/sec, which suggest pressure leak due to rupture of fiber and hence required to be discarded.
  - Total cell volume: It is measured with pushing out of water from the blood compartment with the help of air pushed through syringe. The volume of water coming out is measured. Reduction of TCV below 80% of initial value indicates discarding the dialyser.

- **Automated reprocessing:** In this method returning of blood with heparinized saline and inspection of dialyser remains same as in manual method. The dialyser is connected to the reprocessing machine with appropriate connections of blood and dialysate compartment. The steps of rinsing with water, cleaning with specific chemical agents (commonly 2% peracetic acid), backwashing and tests of performance are carried out in auto mode. If the tests of performance are failed, the dialyser can be discarded. If the test of performance is passed, the printout of the result generated by machine can be taken and to pasted on the dialyser.

SUGGESTED READING

1. Dialyser Reprocessing. Indian J Nephrol. 2020;30(Suppl 1):S38-43. PMID: 33149385; PMCID: PMC7598400.
2. Daugridas JT. Handbook of Dialysis, 5th edition.
3. Nissenson AR. Handbook of dialysis therapy, 1st south Asia edition.

Setting up of Hemodialysis Facility

Rashmi Yadav, Urmila Anandh, Sayali Thakare

INTRODUCTION

Depending on the patient load and hospital setup, the infrastructure for setting up a dialysis unit varies. However, the basic requirements to set up a hemodialysis unit remain the same. In accordance with the recent Indian Hemodialysis guidelines 2020, these requirements can be summarized under following heads:

DIALYSIS AREA

- **Dialysis machines:** Apart from regular hemodialysis machines, separate machines for Hepatis B, Hepatitis C and HIV as per the requirement of the center to be kept in the unit. All machines should with battery backup. Ideally there should also be one stand-by HD machine to be kept for every 10 machines. Similarly, hybrid machines, CRRT machines and Portable RO may also be kept **(Fig. 1)**.
- **Dialysis personnel:** Nephrologist and/or Dialysis Doctor, Technicians, Trained Nurses and Sanitation attendants are required. Access to dietician and medical social worker is desirable.
- **Dialysis area:**
  - Each bed should have minimum area of 11 × 10 feet which should accommodate bed/chair with dialysis machine and some working room. The working room should be sufficient to accommodate two dialysis personnel along with resuscitative equipment when needed. They should be arranged in rows with sufficient space for easy wheel in or out of beds.
  - The beds should have wheels with lock, arrangement for elevation, sitting up and position change. They should be accompanied with a hand rub dispenser at one end and a bed table for patient to eat. Each bed should have a curtain partition for privacy of the patient. Provision for hanging saline bottles and draining used saline should be there near the bed.
  - The unit should be airconditioned.

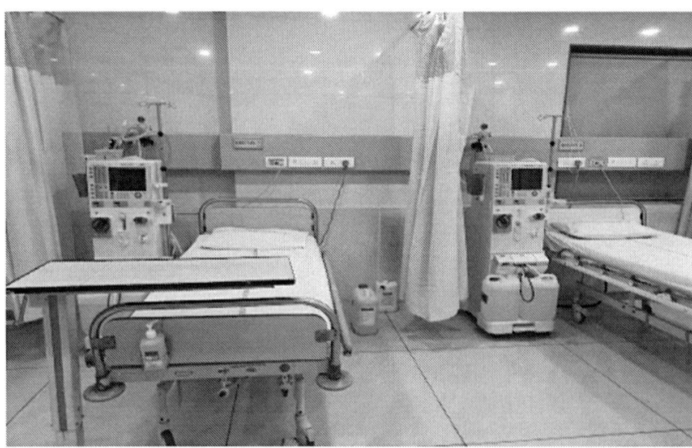

Fig. 1: Dialysis machines.

- Floor should be skid free and easy to maintain, clean and disinfect. Epoxy or vinyl flooring is preferred.
- Walls should be smooth and painted with water resistant washable paint.
- Ceilings should be easily accessible for cleaning. All areas where dust can fall off like pipelines and conduits should have a covered and finished ceiling. Minimum height should be of 2.4–2.7 meters.
- Windows should have washable blinds.
- Natural sunlight access should be maximized.
- Door should be wide enough to allow for trolley bed or wheel chair to enter/exit the unit. Minimum opening width desirable is 1.12 meter.

WATER TREATMENT AND DRAINAGE

- **Area for water treatment and storage:** Water treatment system is the backbone of any dialysis unit. Specified area for RO treatment of municipal water and storage of treated water is a must. The storage tank size can vary upon the number of dialysis beds but it should be in a stainless steel tank with tight fitting lid and tapering bottom for easy disinfection **(Fig. 2)**.
- **Water pipeline system for conveying reverse osmosis (RO) water:** All pipelines should be of medical grade PVC or stainless steel grade 316 material water distribution system should be configured in a loop without dead end or multiple branches. After supplying all machines and reprocessing area, the water line should drain extra RO water back to the RO tank for recirculation **(Fig. 3)**.

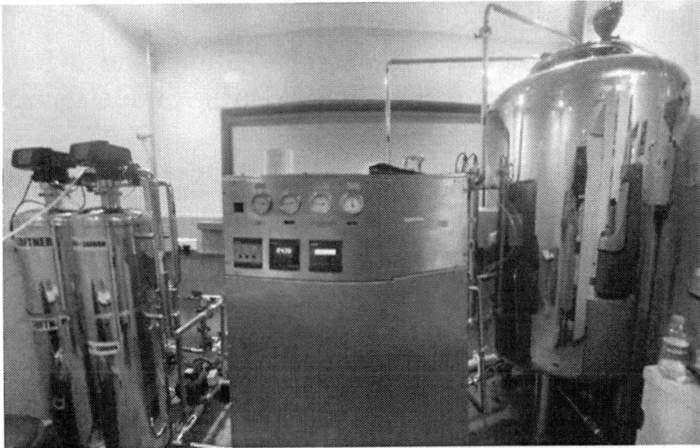

Fig. 2: Water treatment.

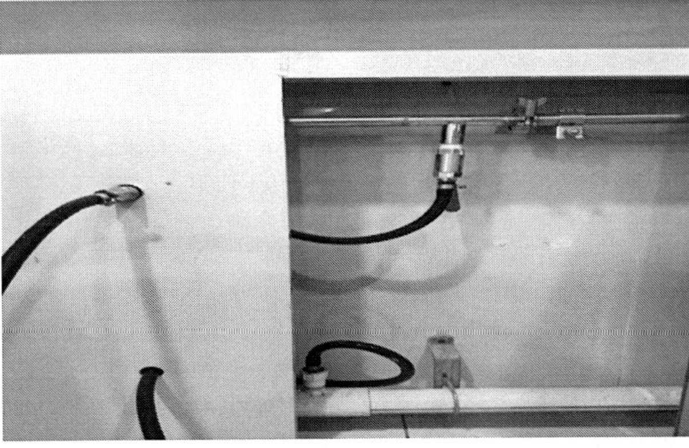

Fig. 3: Water pipeline.

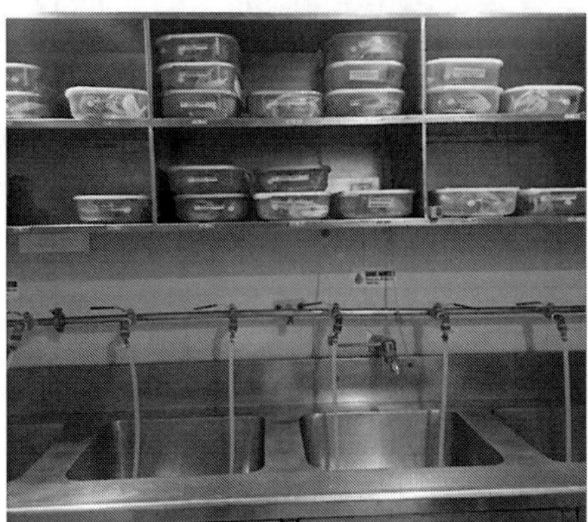

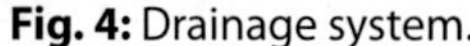
Fig. 4: Drainage system.

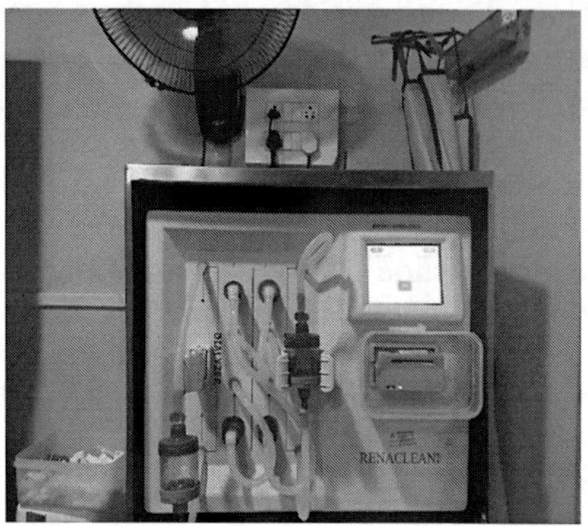

Fig. 5: Electrical and other connections.

- **Drainage system:**
  - High density polyethylene like materials which are chemically resistant should be used in the drainage of dialysate and reprocessing effluent. All drainage line should be connected to the main drainage line without bends or blind end.
  - The highest point in drain pipes should be at least 1–1.5 feet above the floor and downward slope in maintained so lowest point in drain line is 4–6 inches above floor. Regular inspection for mold and proper ventilation is a must **(Fig. 4)**.
- **Electrical and other connections:**
  - At the head end of each bed at least 6 sockets of 5/15 amps should be there for connection of the machine and other equipment. It should also have outlet for oxygen, suction outlet, treated water inlet and a drainage outlet.
  - Minimum 30 minutes backup should be a with a uninterrupted power supply (UPS) or a generator supply line **(Fig. 5)**.

OTHER AREAS

- **Reception area:** An area to receive patients, screen for any febrile/transmittable illness and check vitals. Ideally weighing scale should be near reception to record predialysis weight at the same time.
- **Nursing station:** One or more stations for all round visibility with telecommunication facility and computer access.
- **Isolation room:** Separate area for hepatitis B and hepatitis C patients with independent water supply and drainage facility is desirable (not mandatory) for safety of other patients and staff.
- **Hand washing:**
  - Hand wash basin (one square meter area) made up of steel or porcelain should be there with handle/elbow connector or automatic water flow.
  - Hand rub dispensers to be present at each bedside and at all desirable places.
- **Dialyser reprocessing area:**
  - The number of dialysis machine: sink should be ideally 2:1.
  - At least the washing area should have two sinks with workbench and water pressure of 20 psi. One sink is for initial rinsing of the dialyser and tubing for draining all the blood and for cleansing the dialysate compartment (with treated RO water). The other sink is for filling sterilization agent and labeling.

- Depth of the sink should be atleast 45 cm and a drainage mesh at 20 cm from upper edge, so the dialyser and tubing are in the upper part and not in contact with the lower part which has large opening for removal of used water.
- There should be separate reprocessing unit for HBV and HCV patients.
- Dialyser fiber bundle counting can be done with dialyser reprocessing machine.
- Preparation of bicarbonate solution can be done in the same area with the mixing machine or manually.

❖ **Storage area:**
- Two types—dry storage (new supplies) and Wet storage (reprocessed dialysers and tubing). New supplies include new dialysers and tubing, dry HD concentrate solutions, IV fluids, AV fistula needles, syringes, gloves, sterile trays and other consumables like stationary, records, etc. Reprocessed dialysers and tubing are kept in individual compartments with labeled boxes to avoid mix up.
- Separate workbench for preparation of injection and sterile tray at dialysis start.
- Separate area for clean and dirty utilities.
- At least one refrigerator for storage of injections.

❖ **Emergency cart:** Includes cardiac monitor, pulse oximetry, endotracheal intubation tube, AMBU bag, infusion pump, defibrillator with all emergency medicines should be available in sufficient quantity.

❖ **Weighing scales:** Accurate weighing scale with large platform is a must. Electrical scales or weighing chair for wheel chair bound patient is desirable. Bed with built in weighing scales are required in units using CRRT.

SUPPORT FACILITIES

❖ **Area for record keeping:** A computer-based record keeping is desirable. Hard copy of all dialysis records should be kept and sent to hospital record system as per the hospital norms.

❖ Pest control system and Fire safety system

❖ Toilet

❖ **Duty room:** For nursing staff and technicians to have lockers and to be used as a changing room.

❖ **Audiovisual entertainment:** Television, educational books or magazines may be provided at each bedside and in the waiting room.

❖ **Procedure room:** A 120 square feet room is desirable tor temporary catheter insertion, removal of permanent catheter and other procedures related to hemodialysis. It should have an operating bed, sufficient lights, USG with vascular probe and instrument storage facility. The room can also be multipurpose and can be used for IV medications administration, manage complications postdialysis like high BP, bleeding from AVF, etc., and as a recovery room or consultation room.

❖ **Waiting area:** Outside the HD unit, room for patients awaiting their turn for dialysis and their attendants is required.

❖ **Waste management:** Color coded dustbins is a must for proper disposal of medical waste.

SUGGESTED READING

1. Personnel for Hemodialysis Unit. Indian J Nephrol. 2020;30(Suppl 1):S6-S8.
2. Setting up of Hemodialysis Unit. Indian Journal of Nephrology. 2020;30(Suppl 1):S1-S5.
3. Standard of Care for Maintainance Hemodialysis in India. Ministry of Health and Family Welfare Govt. of India; 2010.

16
CHAPTER

Anticoagulation in Hemodialysis

Asheesh Kumar, Jithu Kurian, Manas Behera

INTRODUCTION

The hemodialysis procedure involves blood remaining in the extracorporeal circuit for 3–4 hours without clotting. This dialysis circuit exhibits variable degrees of thrombogenicity and may initiate blood clotting. To prevent this clotting, we need anticoagulation during hemodialysis.

The visual inspection of the tubing (extremely dark blood), dialyser (shadows of black streak, presence of dark clots at the inflow dialyser head), and drip chamber (foaming with subsequent clot formation) are the various signs suggestive of clotting in the dialysis circuit **(Fig. 1)**. As a result of clotting in the hemodialysis circuit, arterial and venous pressure readings may change depending on the location of the thrombus. The various factors which favor clotting in the extracorporeal circuit are:

- Low blood flow
- High ultrafiltration rate
- Dialysis access recirculation
- Use of drip chamber (air exposure, foam formation and turbulence)
- High hematocrit
- Intradialytic blood product transfusion/lipid infusion

When there is clotting in the dialyser circuit, there is loss of dialyser and blood tubing with loss of approximately 100–180 mL of blood. Unfractionated heparin (UFH) is the most common anticoagulant agent in use. Also, low molecular weight heparin, trisodium citrate, argatroban, heparinoids, and prostanoids may be used as alternative anticoagulants **(Table 1)**.

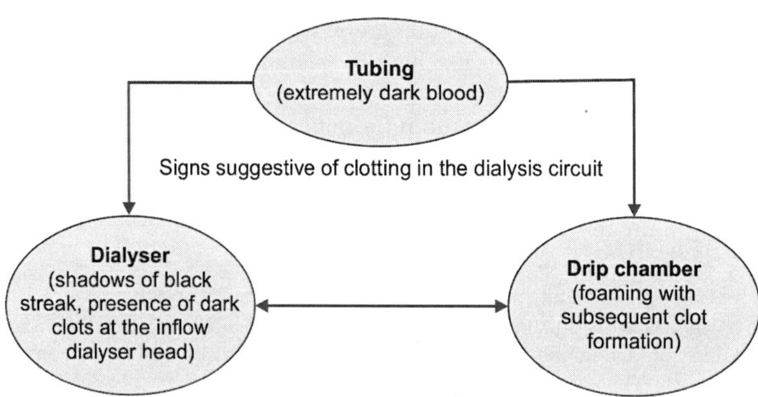

Fig. 1: Visual inspection of clotting.

Table 1: Protocols of various anticoagulants to be used during hemodialysis.

	Dosing protocols			
Anticoagulant	***Loading dose/ bolus***	***Maintenance dose***	***Monitoring***	***Reversal agent***
Unfractionated heparin Standard dose Low dose	2,000–4,000 IU 15–20 IU/kg	500–2,000 IU/h 500 IU/h	aPTT	Protamine sulfate (1 mg/100 IU heparin)
Low molecular weight heparin Enoxaparin	0.50–0.67 mg/kg	NA	Plasma anti-Xa activity	Protamine sulfate (0.5 mg/1 mg enoxaparin)
Regional citrate	NA	100 mL/h trisodium citrate with 35 mmol/h calcium chloride	Ionized calcium Target: Within 10% of baseline level	Calcium chloride

STANDARD HEPARIN DIALYSIS

Heparin changes the conformation of antithrombin, leading to the inactivation of coagulation factors, particularly factor IIa. The commonly used unfractionated heparin preparation is available as 5 mL vials containing 5,000 U/mL (25,000 U/vial). It can be given as an initial bolus dose (2,000 U) via venous access tubing and saline flush. Wait for 3–5 minutes to allow heparin dispersion before initiating dialysis. A constant infusion of 1,200 U/hour follows this through the arterial blood line. Another prescription in the standard dosing is to administer the initial bolus of 4,000 U and then give an additional 1,000–2,000 U bolus dose if necessary. Low-dose protocols, such as 15–20 U/kg loading and 500 U/h maintenance, are also safe and effective. With all protocols, maintenance infusions are typically stopped 60 minutes before the end of dialysis in case of AVF and 30 minutes or can be used till the end of dialysis in case of venous catheters.

Usually, the heparin effect will continue for 6–8 hours after stopping the hemodialysis. Surgical procedures and intramuscular/subcutaneous injections must be avoided during this period. Bleeding, thrombocytopenia, pruritis, anaphylactoid reactions, and hyperkalemia are possible complications. Heparin-induced thrombocytopenia is a complication, is of two types. In Type 1, platelet count decreased to 100 × $10^{12/L}$ within 1–4 days and needs observation, whereas, in Type 2, the platelet count will decrease to 30–50 × $10^{12/L}$. There will be antibody production against the heparin-platelet factor 4 complex, and need nonheparin-based anticoagulation for its management. Heparin rinses followed by saline washout should not be used in these patients.

Heparin therapy is ordinally prescribed empirically without monitoring the coagulation. If required, blood for clotting studies will be withdrawn from the arterial lines proximal to the heparin infusion site.

Low Dose/Tight Heparin

Low dose, also called tight heparin protocols, are used in patients with a high risk of bleeding, which cannot achieve effective HD without anticoagulation. Patients with platelet counts (~75,000–100,000/mm^3), one day before surgery in hemodialysis-dependent patients or up to one week in postoperative patients are commonly practiced indications of tight heparin.

Low Molecular Weight Heparin

A single injection/dose at the start of hemodialysis is sufficient for dialysis treatment. Its use is safe and effective, as evaluated in various long-term studies. High cost and lack of readily available monitoring assays prevent its routine use. Commonly used LMWH compounds are Dalteparin, Enoxaparin, Nadroparin, and Reviparin.

Regional Citrate Anticoagulation (RCA)

Trisodium citrate (500 mmol/L) is infused into the arterial port of the dialysis circuit. Calcium chloride (500 mmol/L) is infused into the venous return before the needle. This can be increased by 2.5–5 mmol/h to keep ICA within 10% of the baseline. This anticoagulation technique is not used regularly for intermittent hemodialysis but for continuous dialysis therapy. The most feared complication of RCA is symptomatic hypocalcemia precipitating cardiac events. The infusion of calcium chloride will neutralize the citrate in the blood before infusion into the patient. This will reduce the risk of citrate-induced hypocalcemia. RCA is primarily metabolized in the liver; there can be a high risk of citrate toxicity and hypocalcemia in severe liver failure, which is an absolute contraindication to RCA.

Heparin Free Dialysis

Heparin rinse of the dialysis circuit with saline containing 3,000 U of heparin/L is optional. Heparin can coat the extracorporeal circuit and mitigate the thrombogenic response. Drain the heparin-containing fluid to prevent systemic heparin administration to the patients. Set the blood flow rate to 300–400 mL/min. There is a need to rinse the dialyser with 250 mL of saline while occluding the blood inlet line every 15 minutes. This frequency of flushes can be increased or decreased according to need. This method is used actively or at high risk of bleeding, pericarditis, thrombocytopenia, or acutely ill patients **(Fig. 2)**.

Heparinoids/Thrombin Inhibitors/Prostanoids

Heparinoids (danaparoid and fondaparinux), Thrombin Inhibitors (argatroban and lepirudin), and prostanoids (prostacyclins and analogs) are also studied in hemodialysis patients, but they are not in regular use.

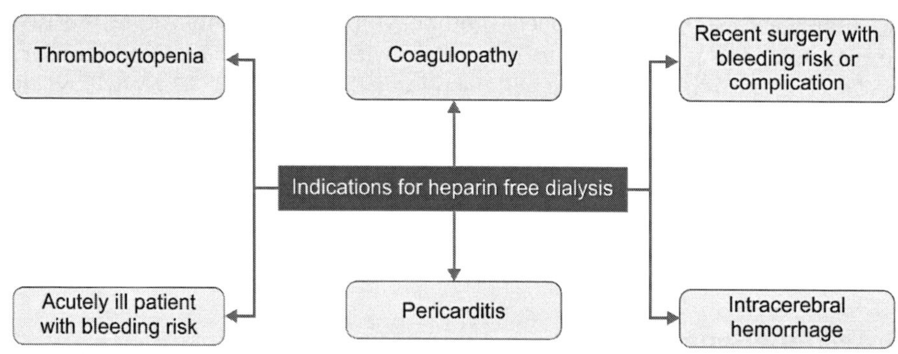

Fig. 2: Heparin free dialysis.

Technical Errors that can Result in Clotting

There may be operator-induced errors that must be considered. If there is a poor priming technique or inadequate priming of the dialysis circuit, the retained air in the dialysis circuit may predispose to clotting. There can be incorrect heparin pump flow rate setting, incorrect loading dose, delayed starting in the heparin pump, failure to release the heparin line clamp, kinking of the outlet bloodline, inadequate blood flow due to needle/catheter positioning or clotting or frequent interruption of blood flow due to machine alarms are the other possible preventable operator induced factors. Protamine sulfate must be in the dialysis facilities if excess heparin is infused accidentally. So, paying attention to these factors can reduce clotting in the dialysis circuit.

SUGGESTED READING

1. Daugirdas JT, Blake PG, Ing TS. Chapter 14: Anticoagulation. In: Handbook of Dialysis, 5th edition. Philadelphia, Penn: Wolters Kluwer. 2014:252-66.
2. Claudel SE, Miles LA, Murea M. Anticoagulation in hemodialysis: A narrative review. In: Seminars in Dialysis. 2021;3(2):103-15.

Monitoring and Management of Dialysis Patient

17 CHAPTER

Asheesh Kumar, Sourabh Sharma, Sambit Sundaray

INTRODUCTION

Dialysis patients are very vulnerable, as there is a need for persistence in care and management. The role of dialysis technicians is vital in the management of these patients. Dialysis technicians spend maximum time with hemodialysis-dependent patients. There are multiple aspects of the patient which need to be observed in each visit. There are some signs, and monitoring these can predict and diagnose the complication early **(Fig. 1)**.

WEIGHT MONITORING

Weight monitoring is of paramount importance in hemodialysis-dependent patients. There is a need to monitor interdialysis weight gain (the difference between the postdialysis weight of the one dialysis and the predialysis weight of the following dialysis) and intradialysis weight loss (weight loss during the dialysis procedure). Dry weight is the ideal postdialysis weight after the removal of all or most of the excess body fluid. Dry weight is the target the clinician prescribes, and dialysis personnel should try and achieve dry weight **(Fig. 2)**.

The maximum ultrafiltration tolerated by the patients is usually 500–700 mL/hour. The weight gain between two dialysis procedures should be 3 kg. If this is above 3 kg, this is suggestive of noncompliance to salt and water. Hypotension, muscle cramps, vomiting, and cardiac events are the possible side effects if the intradialytic weight loss is over 3 kg.

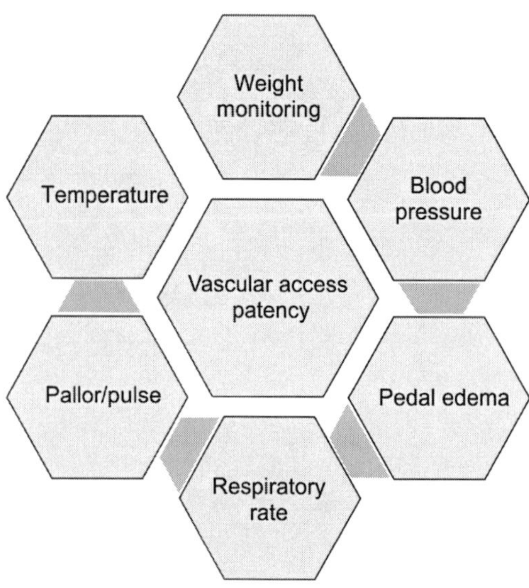

Fig. 1: Monitoring signs of dialysis.

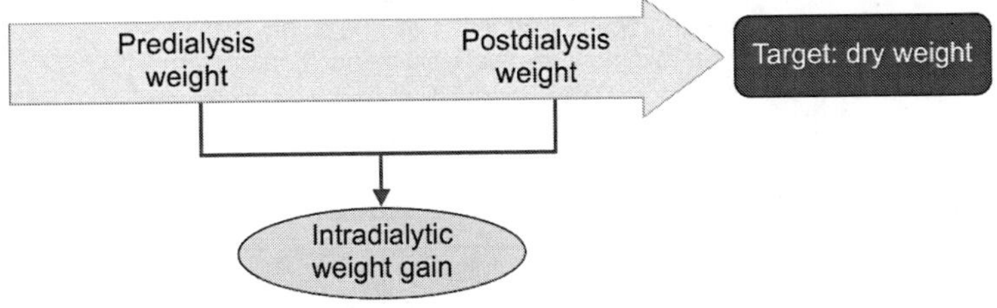

Fig. 2: Weight monitoring.

MONITORING IN DIALYSIS

Blood Pressure

CKD patients usually have high blood pressure, and reasonable control of blood pressure (130 ± 10/90 ± 10 mm Hg) helps to provide adequate and uninterrupted dialysis. Periodic (every 10–15 minutes) blood pressure monitoring is usually done with a hemodialysis machine-built sphygmomanometer. Patients are mainly guided to avoid antihypertensive medication before dialysis. But this dictum is not for all patients. There should be individualization of the treatment for each patient. Blood pressure can increase or decrease during the dialysis treatment. Monitoring of blood pressure during the dialysis will guide.

Temperature

Hemodialysis-dependent patients are at high risk of infection because of their immuno-suppressed state, frequent hospital visits, vascular access (CVCs), and machine exposure. The average temperature of dialysis-dependent patients is also equal to normal healthy persons. A higher body temperature suggests infection, and there is a need to search for the infective foci actively. Patients with CVCs are usually at increased risk of disease and should be monitored for exit site or tunnel infection. The hot feeling during dialysis can also be caused by higher dialysate temperature or as a part of a pyrogen reaction. Regular monitoring of patients and frequent machine checks are also required.

Respiratory Rate

Normal respiratory rate (14–16 per minute) is also a sign of adequate fluid control and good dialysis. Patients on dialysis have a high propensity for breathlessness/dyspnea because of fluid overload (pulmonary edema), associated cardiac failure, or other causes. This also suggests the importance of maintaining the dry weight of the patients. Acute pulmonary edema is a medical emergency and needs immediate dialysis. This will relieve the condition of the patient.

Pallor

Hemodialysis-dependent patients are most of the time anemic. One should regularly monitor this; if severe pallor develops, hemoglobin should be checked before dialysis. Any patient with a hemoglobin level below seven needs a blood transfusion.

Pedal Edema

CKD5 patients are almost in a fluid overload state and have mild pedal edema. Pedal edema should disappear after starting dialysis with ultrafiltration (fluid removal). If a hemodialysis-

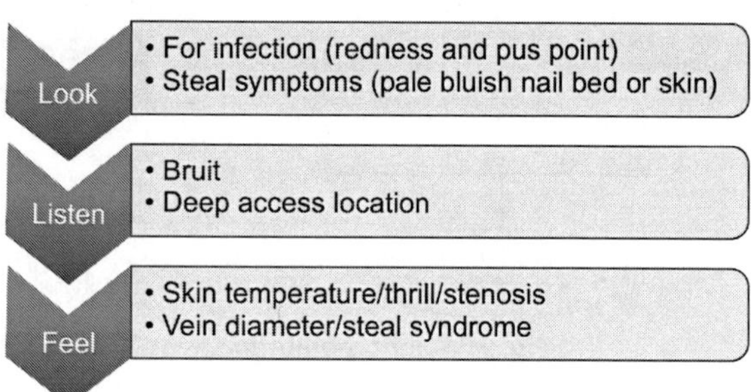

Fig. 3: Arteriovenous fistula monitoring and routine.

dependent patient has pedal edema, it suggests fluid overload that is noncompliance by the patient and inadequate ultrafiltration. This should be managed with a diagnosis and treatment of the cause.

Pulse

Pulse monitoring is also a vital sign and will contribute to diagnosing many issues. An increased heart rate(tachycardia) suggests fever, hypotension, or cardiac problem, whereas an irregular heart rate suggests cardiac problems.

VASCULAR ACCESS

Hemodialysis-dependent patients should be regularly assessed for vascular access. Vascular access is the lifeline for the hemodialysis-dependent patient, and its patency, and adequate blood flow rate, should be assessed periodically. This monitoring is ideally conducted when the patient is not on dialysis. The patient's regular counseling for vascular access care should also be done **(Fig. 3)**.

For arteriovenous fistula monitoring, the routine should be followed as "look, listen, feel and specific tests". One should also look for infection (redness and pus point), steal symptoms (pale bluish nail bed or skin) stenosis (swollen access arm and prominent vein in chest wall). Palpation of thrill, arm elevation test and pulse augmentation test should also be performed regularly for the assessment for AVF which can guide us for inflow or outflow stenosis. In patients with CVCs, exits and tunnel site infection should be checked regularly. Patients with CVCs should also be guided for the preservation/exercise of one limb (venous system) for future AVF creation.

INVESTIGATIONS

Patients on hemodialysis need periodic monitoring by blood investigations. There are guidelines for what are the investigations to be done and how frequently they should be. These are shown in the **Table 1** along with the periodicity. These are done to check the adequacy of the hemodialysis procedure, iron deficiency, treatment, its compliance, and any new infection.

Along with these, there should be record-keeping of each and every patient's vital parameter monitored during the hemodialysis procedure. All adverse effects/complications (dialyser clot/ AV access cannulation complications/CVC dysfunction/any cardiac event or patients having infection) should be noted. Monthly audits of these should be there to identify improvement needs, look for the root cause of the problem and then act on them **(Fig. 4)**.

Table 1: Investigation and periodicity of them.

Periodicity	***Test to be done***
Every 2 weeks	Hemoglobin
Monthly	Complete blood count, serum albumin, blood urea nitrogen, creatinine, calcium, magnesium, phosphorus, glucose, sodium, potassium, transferrin saturation HBV, HCV, HIV
Every 3 months	Serum ferritin and plasma intact parathyroid hormone
When needed	Blood culture

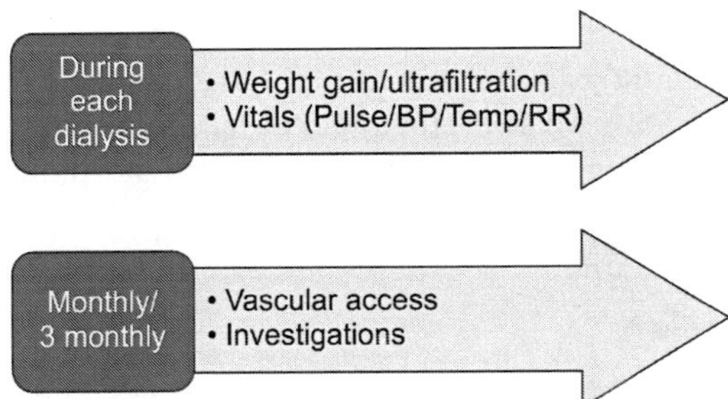

Fig. 4: Patient's vital parameter monitored.

SUGGESTED READING

1. Daugirdas JT, Blake PG, Ing TS. Chapter 14: anticoagulation. In: Handbook of Dialysis, 5th edition. Philadelphia, Penn: Wolters Kluwer; 2014.
2. Lok CE, Huber TS, Lee T, Shenoy S, Yevzlin AS, Abreo K, et al. KDOQI Vascular Access Guideline Work Group. KDOQI clinical practice guideline for vascular access: 2019 update. Am J Kidney Dis. 2020;75(4) (suppl 2):S1-164.

Complications During Hemodialysis

Mohan V Bhojaraja, Dharshan Rangaswamy, Jyothipriya Jyothindrakumar

INTRODUCTION

Patients undergoing hemodialysis may encounter various complications throughout the procedure. These complications can be incapacitating, potentially fostering resistance to dialysis and thereby contributing to increased mortality and morbidity.

COMMON COMPLICATIONS

Intradialytic Hypotension

- **Defined** as a nadir (lowest) SBP <90 mm Hg (most accepted), seen in 5–30% of all dialysis treatments and risk factors being old age, diabetes, low albumin, lower predialysis BP, females and longer vintage.
- **Causes** include volume related-large weight gain, short dialysis time, low target ("dry") weight; inadequate vasoconstriction-high dialysate temperature, autonomic neuropathy, antihypertensives, eating during treatment anemia; cardiac factors and rarely hemorrhage, sepsis, dialyser reaction, hemolysis and air embolism.
- **Management**: Ultrafiltration should be stopped → position the patient in the trendelenburg position → administer IV fluid bolus (rapid administration of hypertonic saline or slow administration of 0.9% saline).
- **Preventive strategies**:
  1. *First-line approach*: Review the dry weight assessment, adjust the timing of antihypertensive medications, refrain from food intake during dialysis, ensure dialysate calcium and magnesium levels are at or above 2.25 mEq/L and 1.0 mEq/L, respectively, restrict interdialytic sodium intake, and reconsider the dialysate sodium prescription.
  2. *Second-line approach*: Evaluate cardiac function, increase the dialysis treatment time and use cool-temperature dialysate.
  3. *Third-line approach*: Midodrine (2.5–5 mg, prior to dialysis), change to other modes of dialysis, and correction of anemia.

Intradialytic Hypertension

- **Major cause** for intradialytic hypertension is volume expansion, although sympathetic overactivity and activation of the renin-angiotensin system also contribute.
- For patients on dialysis, we use self-recorded home BP. If not possible, midweek median intradialytic systolic BP is used, with a target of <140/80 mm Hg.
- **Management**: Reduce target dry weight, start treatment with beta blocker followed by addition of other antihypertensive medications.

Chest Pain

- Mild chest pain is seen in 1–4% of dialysis with no known cause and no specific treatment.
- **Management:** Stop ultrafiltration → decrease the blood flow rate to equal or less than 200 mL/min → place the patient in a supine position → administer oxygen → document vital signs → visually examine the venous line blood for air bubbles or a port-wine appearance → obtain a 12-lead electrocardiogram → if persistent chest pain, then dialysis should be discontinued.

Dialyser Reactions

Type A reactions (less common): Seen in first few minutes. Mild symptoms include urticaria, cough, wheezing, headache, nausea, vomiting. Severe reactions include hypotension, dyspnea and potentially resulting in cardiac arrest and death.

- Can be **due to** ethylene oxide, AN69-associated reactions, dialysate contamination, reuse heparin and complement fragment release.
- **Management** involves discontinuing dialysis and implementing supportive therapies, such as antihistamines, steroids, and epinephrine.
- **Prevention:** Rinsing of the dialyser, employing effective sterilization techniques, refraining from dialyser reuse, and avoiding the use of polyacrylonitrile (PAN) membranes in patients undergoing ACE inhibitor treatment.

Type B reactions: Occur 15–30 minutes into the dialysis, often improves with continuation of the dialysis. The most common symptoms are dyspnea, nausea, vomiting chest and back pain. They are complement mediated. The treatment is supportive and can be prevented by reuse of the dialyser.

Cramps

- It's a common complication the pathogenesis of which is unknown. The most common causes include hypotension, hypovolemia, high ultrafiltration rate, and use of low-sodium dialysate.
- **Prevention:** Stretching exercises, adjusting dialysate sodium and magnesium, use of biotin, carnitine, oxazepam, vitamin E and quinine.
- **Management:** Treatment with 0.9% saline, hypertonic solutions (saline, glucose and mannitol)

Seizures

- Seizures may result from diverse factors including uremic encephalopathy, dialysis disequilibrium syndrome (DDS), hemodynamic instability during dialysis, dialysis dementia associated with aluminum exposure, air embolism, hypoglycemia, hypocalcemia, and hyponatremia.
- **Emergency intervention** involves discontinuing dialysis and ensuring patient safety. Serum levels of glucose and other electrolytes should be assessed and appropriately adjusted.

Dialysis Disequilibrium Syndrome

DDS is characterized by neurological symptoms affecting patients initiating hemodialysis or those who have missed multiple consecutive sessions.

Risk factors: Elevated blood urea nitrogen (BUN) levels (>175 mg/dL or 60 mmol/L), extremes of age, pre-existing neurologic diseases, encephalitis, and cerebral edema.

Pathogenesis: Cerebral edema is theorized to be induced by the rapid clearance of urea and other osmoles during hemodialysis, resulting in a swift decline in plasma osmolality and subsequent water movement into neurons.
Clinical manifestations: Restlessness, progressing to confusion, headache, nausea, blurred vision, disorientation, seizures, coma, mania, and potential fatality.
Prevention: For newly initiated hemodialysis patients, commence with short sessions at low blood flow and sodium modeling may be employed for patients with recurrent nonadherence.
Treatment: Halt dialysis and investigate alternative causes. If severe DDS persists despite sodium modeling, consider a trial of hypertonic saline or mannitol. Subsequently, plan for daily, short, low-efficiency dialysis sessions akin to the initiation phase for new dialysis patients.

Headache, Nausea, and Vomiting

- These are nonspecific common symptoms usually in which dialysis is continued, antiemetics and supportive treatment are given.
- **Syndrome of dialysis-associated headache:** Either bifrontal or temporal following dialysis commencement, intensifying throughout the session, and resolving within 72 hours which is attributed to alterations in vasoactive nitric oxide.

Hemolysis

- May be a medical emergency manifested by back pain, tightness in the chest, and shortness of breath with dramatic deepening of skin pigmentation and port-wine appearance of blood in the venous blood line.
- Seen with an obstruction in the blood line and issue with dialysis solution.
- **Management:** Stop blood pump immediately and clamp the blood lines → Severe hyperkalemia may occur, and this may require additional dialysis/antihyperkalemic measures

Air Embolism

- Is a possible disaster that, if not identified and handled promptly, can be fatal.
- **Symptoms:** Dyspnea, cough, chest tightness, loss of consciousness, convulsions, and even death.
- **Identification:** Foam is often seen in the venous blood line of the dialyser and churning sound may be heard on auscultation.
- **Management:** Clamp the venous blood line and stop the blood pump → recumbent position on the left side with the chest and head tilted downward → cardiorespiratory support.

SUGGESTED READING

1. Bagdasarian N, Heung M, Malani PN. Infectious complications of dialysis access devices. Infect Dis Clin North Am. 2012;26(1):127-41.
2. Saha M, Allon M. Diagnosis, Treatment, and Prevention of Hemodialysis Complications. Clin J Am Soc Nephrol. 2017;12(2):357-69.

Infections in Dialysis Patients

19
CHAPTER

Jai Inder Singh, Indranil Ghosh, Shyam Bihari Bansal

INTRODUCTION

Infection is the second most leading cause of hospital admission and death in dialysis patients. Dialysis patients are at higher risk of infections than healthy population due to poor immunity and malnutrition.

The most common infections in dialysis patients are:

- Catheter-related blood stream infection (CRBSI)
- Infected AV graft or fistula
- CAPD peritonitis
- **Community acquired infections:** Pneumonia, UTI and TB

The factors contributing to the increase in risk of infections are as given in **Figure 1**.

The potential sources of infection in a dialysis patient are as given in **Table 1**.

Catheter-related Blood Stream Infections

The catheter is a foreign body and becomes a source of infection if used for a long time. The bacteria can enter the blood via skin contamination or through the catheter hub **(Fig. 2)**. It is defined as blood culture positive infection after 48 hours of catheter insertion. The infection can spread to other parts of the body (vertebra, heart valves, etc.). Dialysis staff need to be aware of ways to prevent CRBSI **(Table 2)**.

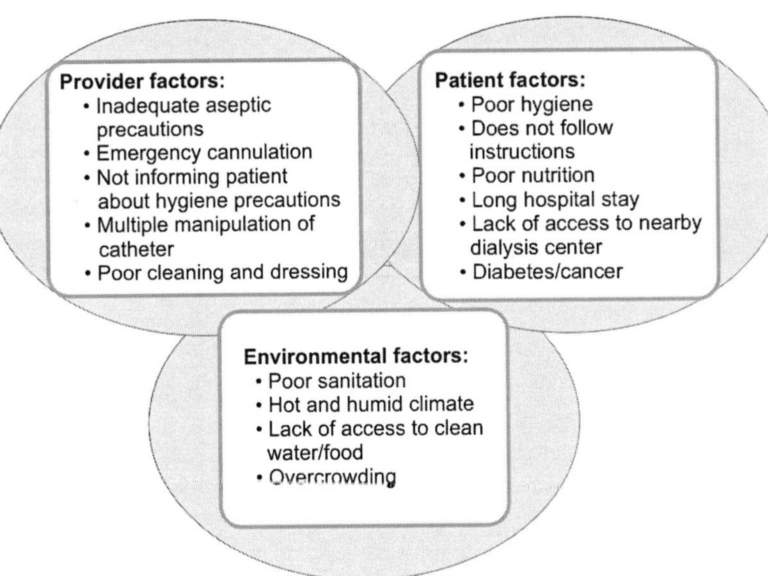

Fig. 1: Factors contributing to risk of infection in dialysis patients.

Table 1: Potential sources of infection in a dialysis patient.

Sl. No.	*Hemodialysis*	*Remarks*
1.	Non tunneled catheter (DLJC/DLFC)	CRBSI (bacteria from skin/catheter hub)
2.	Tunnelled catheter (permanent catheter)	
3.	AV graft	Graft infection
4.	AV fistula	Skin infection over fistula site
5.	RO water contamination	Lack of RO plant maintenance
6.	Dialysate contamination	During bicarbonate preparation manually
7.	Dialyser reuse	Unhygienic storage
8.	IV fluid contamination	During dialyser priming and rinsing
9.	Contaminated hands	Lack of proper hand hygiene
10.	Dialysis machine	Lack of cleaning/disinfection protocol
Peritoneal dialysis		
CAPD catheter exit site infection/peritonitis		Improper exit site care and hand hygiene

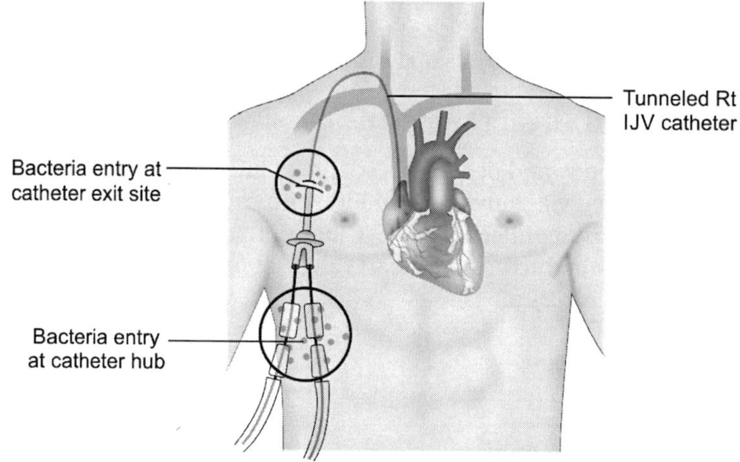

Fig. 2: Portal of entry for microbes—central catheter.

Table 2: Measures to prevent CRBSI.

1.	Follow checklist for catheter insertion
2.	Perform hand hygiene
3.	Prophylactic IV antibiotic (Vancomycin) 1 hour before procedure
4.	Use of alcoholic chlorhexidine for skin preparation
5.	Use of chlorhexidine dressing
6.	Use of antibiotic impregnated catheters
7.	Clean the hub and caps with alcohol/chlorhexidine for 15 seconds before use
8.	Regular change of dressing
9.	Patient education on care of catheter
10.	Dialysis machine

Fever and chills during or after dialysis is the most common feature of CRBSI. Blood culture sample from the catheter should be taken before starting IV antibiotic. Nontunnelled catheter should be removed as early as possible to avoid sepsis. Heparin lock with antibiotic may be used for tunnelled catheter infection.

The choice of antibiotics used in CRBSI are based on the culture sensitivity. However antibiotics like inj Vancomycin or inj teicoplanin (Antistaphylocaccal antibiotic), aminoglycosides like amikacin or netilmycin (for gram negative organisms) or broad spectrum antibiotics like ceftazidime or meropenem may be used, as empirical choices, based on the dialysis center protocol.

RO Water Contamination

During dialysis, HD patients are exposed to large amounts of water coming in contact with blood across the dialyser membrane. When the water treatment system fail, or there is significant contamination, the product water may be unsuitable for dialysis. Water treatment systems and HD machines are susceptible to growth of Gram-negative bacteria and nontuberculous mycobacteria. Gram-negative bacteria also produce endotoxins. It can cause fever, chills, hypotension, headache, and muscle ache occurring during dialysis or within a few hours after dialysis. Endotoxin is removed by reverse osmosis and by endotoxin filters. **Table 3** lists measures to prevent RO water contamination.

Prevention of Transmissible Infections

HIV, HBV and HCV are infections spread through blood. Air borne infections like COVID 19 and TB can also occur with close contact. Strict adherence to universal precautions like hand hygiene and wearing PPE during procedures and hemodialysis is key to prevention **(Table 4)**. Surface disinfection with 1% sodium hypochlorite and heat disinfection of dialysis machine after every dialysis should be done.

Table 3: Steps to avoid RO water contamination.

1.	Avoid prolonged storage of RO water in tanks
2.	Regular cleaning and changing of RO membrane
3.	Avoid very long loops and too many bends in pipeline
4.	Regular disinfection of the RO pipes
5.	Regular testing of RO water quality

Table 4: Steps to prevent transmissible infections.

1.	Consider all patients and surfaces to be potentially infected
2.	Don't recap or reuse needles and syringes
3.	Perform hand hygiene and wear new gloves for each patient
4.	Prepare IV injections separately for each patient at a dedicated station for the purpose
5.	Do not take same vial/syringe or tray to other patients
6.	Use color coded biowaste disposal dustbin for waste disposal
7.	Use barrier precautions for potentially infected patients like COVID
8.	Avoid carrying dialyser and tubing for reprocessing without plastic bag

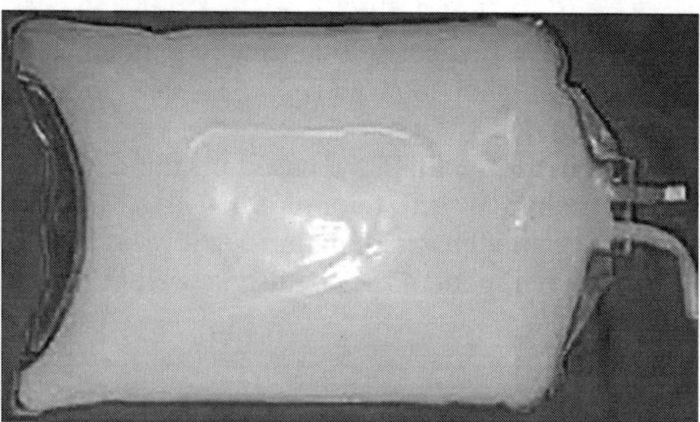

Fig. 3: Show turbid CAPD fluid in CAPD peritonitis.

Infection in CAPD Patients

CAPD catheter is inserted into the abdomen for peritoneal dialysis. It can be a source of infection spreading into the peritoneum causing CAPD peritonitis if not handled in a aseptic manner. The infections associated with CAPD catheter are:

- Exit site infection
- CAPD catheter tunnel infection
- CAPD peritonitis

CAPD peritonitis may be diagnosed with symptoms of fever and abdominal pain, turbid PD fluid **(Fig. 3)**, and CAPD fluid evaluation showing increased cells (>100/cumm) with a positive CAPD fluid culture. It may be treated with intraperitoneal or intravenous antibiotics-based on culture reports, with the choice of empirical antibiotic being Inj vancomycin with a third-generation cephalosporin/aminoglycoside. Refractory cases, resistant cases, fungal or TB peritonitis may require removal of the CAPD catheter.

Exit site infection is defined as the presence of purulent discharge at the catheter and skin junction. Exit site infection may be treated with antibiotics-based on culture sensitivity of discharge/pus.

Measures to prevent infection are:

- Proper hand hygiene before touching catheter
- Drying of exit site with clean cloth after bath
- Application of antiseptic (mupirocin) ointment around exit site
- Avoid pulling the catheter
- Avoid swimming in dirty water
- Control of blood sugar if diabetic

SUGGESTED READING

1. Farrington CA, Allon M. Management of the hemodialysis patient with catheter-related bloodstream infection. Clinical Journal of the American Society of Nephrology. 2019;14(4):611-3.
2. Greenberg KI, Choi MJ. Hemodialysis Emergencies: Core Curriculum 2021. American Journal of Kidney Diseases. W.B. Saunders, 2021;77. p. 796–809.
3. O'Grady NP. Prevention of Central Line–Associated Bloodstream Infections. In: Taichman DB (Ed). New England Journal of Medicine [Internet]. 2023;389(12):1121-31. Available from: http://www.nejm.org/doi/10.1056/NEJMra2213296
4. Sarnak MJ, Jaber BL. Mortality caused by sepsis in patients with end-stage renal disease compared with the general population. Kidney Int. 2000;58(4).

20
CHAPTER

Hemodiafiltration

Rashmi Yadav, Narinder Pal Singh, Harbir Singh Kohli

INTRODUCTION

Hemodiafiltration is a modality to have better convective clearance of uremic toxins especially the middle molecules. It is a combination of hemodialysis and hemofiltration.

BASICS OF HEMODIAFILTRATION (HDF)

It works on two types of mechanism—diffusion and convection. When blood and dialysate pass in opposite directions inside the dialyser, across a semipermeable membrane, small solutes (urea, creatinine, potassium, bicarbonate, etc.) are exchanged based on concertation gradient. This is diffusion which is inversely related to the molecular weight. Hence, larger molecules like beta-2 microglobulin have slow to nil clearance in hemodialysis. However, in convection, two things are different. First, a high flux dialyser membrane is used which can transport large sized solutes across them. Second, replacement fluid is added in the blood compartment for more ultrafiltration. So apart from diffusion taking place between the blood and dialysate compartments, there is solvent drag from the blood to dialysate compartment as shown in **Figure 1**. This bulk fluid flow irrespective of the molecular weight helps in clearance of uremic toxins of middle and large molecular weight.

Convective clearance depends on two things—sieving coefficient and total ultrafiltered volume. Sieving coefficient varies for different membranes and different solutes, while total ultrafiltrate refers to total fluid removed during the treatment plus the replacement or the substitution fluid given during the treatment for increasing convection. Replacement fluid can be pre-prepared sterile fluid from a pharmacy or prepared by the dialysis machine. HDF is costly compared to regular hemodialysis and requires sophisticated machines.

Technical Requirements

- Good vascular access which delivers blood flow rate of at least 350–400 mL/min in the machine.

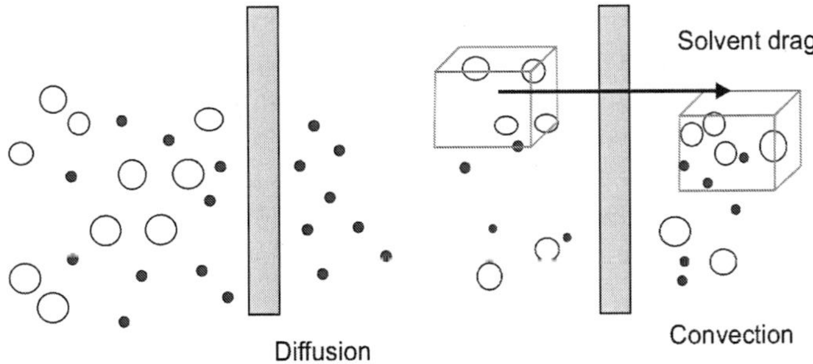

Fig. 1: Basics of hemodiafiltration.

- High flux hemodiafilter which has water permeability of at least (KUF) >20 mL per hour per mm Hg, solute permeability (sieving coefficient of Beta-2 microglobulin) >0.6 and surface area 1.6–1.8 m^2. It is also desirable to have fiber bundle length <30 cm and internal fiber diameter >200 micrometer for low internal blood resistance and better ultrafiltration.
- Machines with online HDF which produce replacement fluid from dialysate fluid using two endotoxin filters. The endotoxin filters need to be disinfected within the machine after each dialysis session and are replaced periodically (either after specified duration of use or number of sessions).
- Ultrapure water with stringent criteria of purity for sterile and nonpyrogenic fluid. Basic requirement includes pretreatment with two RO modules in series and ultrafilters within the hemodiafiltration machine.

The following **Table 1** highlights the differences between various dialysis modalities:

Table 1: Differences between various dialysis modalities.

Parameters	***Hemodialysis***	***Hemofiltration***	***Hemodiafiltration***
Principle	Diffusion	Convection	Diffusion + convection
Dialyser	Low or high flux	High flux	High flux
Blood flow	250–400 mL/min	350–400 mL/min	350–400 mL/min
Dialysate flow	500–800 mL/min	Nil	500–800 mL/min
Replacement fluid	Not required	Required	Required
Cost	Relatively cheap	Costly	Most costly
Uremic toxin removal	Low molecular weight	Middle molecule	Middle molecule
India	Most common	Least common	Increasing use
Endotoxin filter in situ machine	No	Yes	Yes

HDF PRESCRIPTION

Generally, 4 hours HDF session three times a week is prescribed to most patients. More extended and more frequent session as per need can be done.

- **Ultrafiltration (UF):** Greater UF is achieved by adding replacement fluid to blood compartment in 3 ways. If it enters arterial line before entering the dialyser it is called predilution mode **(Fig. 2A)**, if it enters the system after blood passes through the dialyser, it is called postdilution mode **(Fig. 2B)**. It can also be mixed mode where pre and postdilution both are there**(Fig. 2C)**. Based on it, total volume varies. Most commonly used mode is postdilution mode as it gives the most solute clearance. Target UF should be 85–90 mL/kg per hour (20–24 liters approximately). If its predilution mode, target UF should be multiplied by 2 and if its mixed dilution mode then UF should be multiplied by 1.3.
- **Anticoagulation:** HDF requires higher anticoagulation compared to normal dialysis. Heparin bolus should be given in venous needle or blood line and allow to mix in patient blood for 3–5 minutes before entering machine system. It should not be given as a bolus into the hemodiafilter inlet as 50% of unfractionated and 80% of low molecular weight heparin will be lost due to first pass effect as it is unbound to blood proteins.

Advantages of HDF

- **Better clearance of solutes:**
  - 30–40% more Beta-2 microglobulin clearance than high flux hemodialysis.

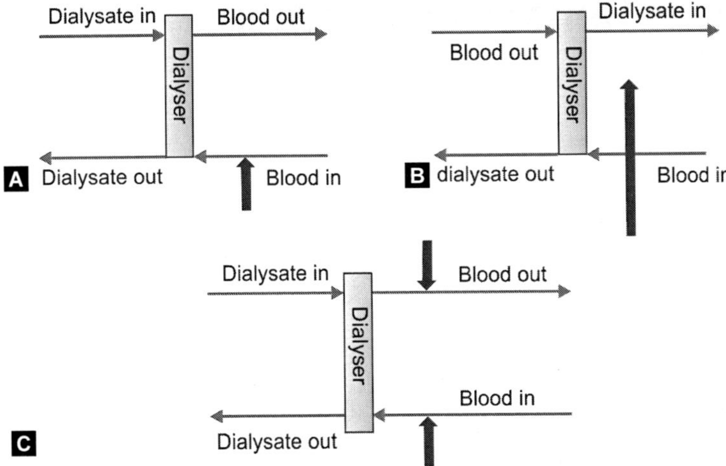

Figs. 2A to C: (A) Predilution substitution fluid; (B) Postdilution substitution fluid; (C) Pre- and postdilution substitution fluid.

- 15–20% more phosphorus clearance.
- Removal of FGF 23, complement factor D, Leptin, various cytokines and erythropoiesis inhibitors, immunoglobulin light chains and advanced glycation end products.

❖ **Clinical benefits:**
- Less intradialytic hypotension.
- Better preservation of residual renal function and patient maintains urine output for longer duration.
- Lesser dose of erythropoietin.
- Better appetite and nutritional status.
- Better dyslipidemia control and prevention of atherosclerosis.
- Lesser incidence of carpal tunnel syndrome.

❖ Longer survival and lesser cardiovascular morbidity is noted when higher UF volumes are done.

Cautions While HDF

❖ Regular water quality check is very important. Failure of cold sterilization or inadequate disinfection can lead to serious side effects. Regular blood CRP check is a good practice in HDF patients.

❖ Increase protein loss can happen due to high flux dialyser hence good supplementation along with dietary protein is required.

❖ Supplementation of various multivitamins and trace elements which are lost during HDF is necessary.

❖ The rate of UF should be restricted to 25–30% of blood flow rate as higher UF can cause dialyser clotting due to hemoconcentration.

SUGGESTED READING

1. Bernard C, Sudhir B, Stefano S. Hemodiafiltration, Handbook of Dialysis, 5th edition. Chapter 17, 321-32.
2. Canaud B, Vienken J, Ash S, Ward RA. Kidney Health Initiative HDF Workgroup: Hemodiafiltration to Address Unmet Medical Needs ESKD Patients. Clin J Am Soc Nephrol. 2018;13(9):1435-43.
3. Francisco M. Hemodiafiltration Hemodialysis International 2005;9:47-55.

Continuous Renal Replacement Therapy

21
CHAPTER

Vishal Singh, Vineet Behera, Dinesh Khullar

INTRODUCTION

The choice of renal replacement therapy (RRT) modality for acute kidney injury (AKI) includes intermittent hemodialysis (IHD) or hybrid therapy, peritoneal dialysis (PD) and continuous renal replacement therapy (CRRT). Many patients hospitalized in the intensive care unit are hemodynamically unstable and have multiorgan failure. Although the choice of RRT in such a setting is determined by the availability of equipment and trained manpower, when available CRRT is considered the gold standard. In CRRT, the rate of fluid and solute removal is slow, and hence fewer episodes of hypotension.

Benefits of CRRT

- **Acid-base, electrolyte and fluid homeostasis**: By providing a slow continuous exchange of solute it maintains the body's homeostasis.
- **Hemodynamic stability:** Unlike HD, fluid removal is slow allowing the filling of intravascular compartments from adjoining tissue and hence well tolerated.
- **Fluid removal:** It very efficiently removes the excess fluid in conditions like ARDS and pulmonary edema.
- **Allows administration of drugs, fluid and total parenteral nutrition:** The excess fluid required to be administered is removed by the machine, preventing fluid overload.
- **Removing uremic toxins**
- **User-friendly machine**

TYPES OF CRRT

The solute is removed by either diffusion or convection or both based on CRRT modality as shown in **Figure 1**.

1. **Continuous venovenous hemofiltration (CVVH):** Based on the principle of convection, it uses hydrostatic pressure to induce ultrafiltration. A dialysis solution is not used. As the ultrafiltration is high, it requires commensurate replacement fluid.
2. **Continuous venovenous hemodialysis (CVVHD):** Based on diffusion, it works like intermittent HD with countercurrent flow of dialysate and blood.
3. **Continuous venovenous hemodiafiltration (CVVHDF):** It combines diffusion with convection and requires both dialysate and replacement fluid.
4. **Slow continuous ultrafiltration (SCUF):** It is based solely on convection and is used to treat isolated fluid overload. No replacement fluid is required.

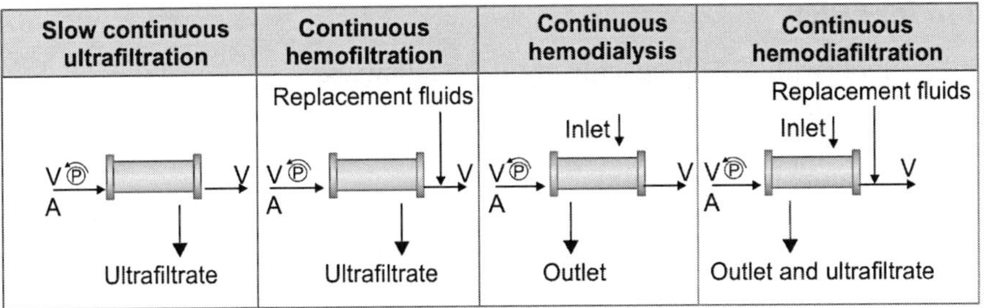

Fig. 1: Continuous renal replacement therapy.

CRRT TECHNIQUE

Access

1. **Access:** Double lumen catheter placed in the internal jugular vein (IJV) or the femoral vein (FV)
2. **Catheter size:** 11–12 Fr catheter of correct length; right IJV-15 cm, left IJV-18 cm and FV-25 cm
3. **Catheter change schedule:** Change only when clinically indicated, i.e., it has either been blocked or is infected

Access Machine (Fig. 2)

The equipment may vary from model to model, but the basic components are similar.

- Roller pumps for blood and dialysate
- Mechanism for ultrafiltration control
- An LCD monitor displays the parameter setting
- Substitution and dialysate heater
- Monitoring system for arterial and venous pressure, blood leak detector, etc.

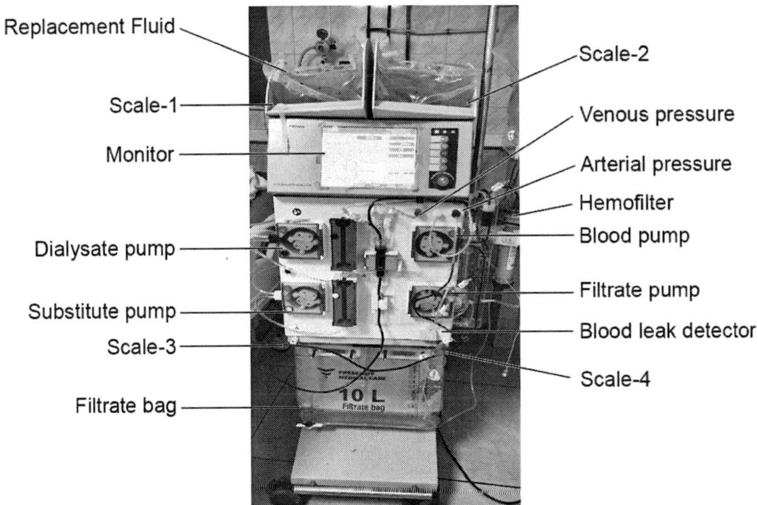

Fig. 2: Machine for continuous renal replacement therapy. *(For color version, see Plate 8)*

Indication for CRRT

Critically ill patients with AKI along with any of the following:
- Refractory hyperkalemia
- Fluid overload unresponsive to optimal medical care
- Uremic encephalopathy, pericarditis
- Severe acidosis refractory to medical therapy (pH <7.2)
- Situations where CRRT is better than HD or PD for RRT
  - Acute brain injury or other causes of increased intracranial pressure.
  - Drug toxicity with dialyzable agents but with slow transportation from the extravascular to the vascular compartment.
  - Hemodynamically unstable patients requiring large volume fluid administration.

Consumables Required

1. **Tubing** is machine-specific. The arterial segment has a port for anticoagulation and predilution replacement. The venous segment has a sampling port and a port for post-dilution replacement fluid.
2. **Hemofilter:** Biocompatible high permeability, high flux membrane
3. **Replacement fluid:** It is a commercially available fluid to replace the fluid removed. It is sterile, pyrogen-free, and contains the buffer (bicarbonate or lactate-based) and electrolytes.
4. **Anticoagulation:** To prevent clotting inside the circuit.
   - *Regional citrate-based:* The citrate chelates the calcium and thus impairs coagulation. A large part of calcium citrate is filtered out in the affluent and those which return to the body are metabolized by the liver. The major complication is hypocalcemia.
   - *Systemic unfractionated heparin (common):*
     - Inject 2,000–5,000 units of heparin in the patient's venous line for systemic anticoagulation
     - Constant infusion of 500–1,000 units/hour through infusion pump into arterial line till CRRT is being performed.
     - Monitor APTT, and keep arterial APTT between 40 and 45 by increasing or decreasing heparin by 100 IU/hr.
   - *No anticoagulation:* Performed by rinsing the circuit with 500 mL saline every 30 minutes. The risk of circuit clotting will increase.

Goal of Therapy

- Maintain fluid balance
- Maintain acid-base and electrolytes
- Avoid complications of uremia
- Maintain function of kidneys

Therapy Dose

The dose is based on the effluent flow rate. The target is 25 mL/kg/hour so that despite downtime or interruption in therapy we achieve at least 20 mL/kg/hour over 24 hours. The total effluent is based on the therapy being performed.
- **CVVH:** It is ultrafiltrate volume
- **CVVHD:** Spend dialysate + ultrafiltrate
- **CVVHDF:** Spend dialysate+ ultrafiltrate + replacement fluid

COMPLICATIONS OF CRRT

- **Hypotension:** Especially when net ultrafiltration is high or in those with diabetic neuropathy
- **Infection:** Usually catheter-related bloodstream infection
- **Bleeding:** Anticoagulant-related
- Hypothermia
- **Electrolyte imbalance:**
  - Hypophosphatemia (incidence >50%; consequences–prolonged respiratory failure)
  - Hypokalemia
  - Hypomagnesemia
  - Hypocalcemia
- **Acid-base imbalance:** Alkalosis with citrate anticoagulation

Common Troubleshooting

- **Signs of hemofilter clotting:** If there is a significant fall in blood flow and the blood in the circuit appears dark in color, suspect clotting. The majority of clotting starts in the venous air trap and not the hemofilter. If this occurs, the circuit needs to be changed.
- **Microbubble introduction and blockage of hemofilter:** Microbubbles are introduced during the priming so be liberal while priming the circuit.
- **Regional citrate anticoagulation:** If the patient develops muscle cramps, tetany, seizures or numbness around the mouth suspect hypocalcemia and replace intravenous calcium gluconate.

SUGGESTED READING

1. Karkar A, Ronco C. Prescription of CRRT: A pathway to optimize therapy. Ann Intensive Care. 2020;10:32.
2. Tandukar S, Palevsky PM. Continuous Renal Replacement Therapy: Who, When, Why, and How. Chest. 2019;155(3):626-38.

Therapeutic Plasma Exchange

22
CHAPTER

Sumita Bhogal, T Murari, Priti Meena

DEFINITION

Plasmapheresis is defined as automated selective removal of plasma. Therapeutic plasma exchange (TPE) is defined as removal of patient's plasma and replacement with other physiological fluids. It is an extracorporeal treatment designed for the removal of plasma along with pathogenic substances such as antibodies, immune complexes or large molecular weight substances from the plasma.

Principle

At least one of the following should be present for TPE to be indicated:
- Sufficiently large molecule
- Long half life
- Acutely toxic substance
- Low volume of distribution

1–1.5 Plasma volume equivalents are exchanged during a plasmapheresis session. Largest decrease occurs with removal of the first plasma volume. Removal of subsequent plasma volumes during same session becomes progressively less effective in decreasing the concentration of the molecule.

Plasma volume is calculated using Kaplan formula

Kaplan formula: For estimated plasma volume = 0.07 × wt (kg) × (1-hct)*

*Hct: Hematocrit

METHODS AND PROCEDURE

TPE is usually performed using either centrifugation or membrane methods. Both have their own advantages and disadvantages. The former separated the plasma from cellular components-based on density and the latter separates plasma-based on molecular size.

Centrifugal TPE (Fig. 1)

Whole blood is pumped into a separation chamber rotating at a high speed and components are separated into layers-based upon their density. The plasma layer is removed and discarded and remaining cellular elements are mixed with a replacement fluid and returned back to the patient. Anticoagulant usually citrate is added before centrifugation and spun at a speed of 200–2,500 rpm.

Centrifugation is usually of two types (Table 1): Intermittent vs continuous apheresis.

Membrane TPE (Fig. 2)

Plasma filter membrane allows plasma, proteins and pathogens to pass through and can be discarded. Platelets and cells are retained. Substitution fluid is added and the processed blood

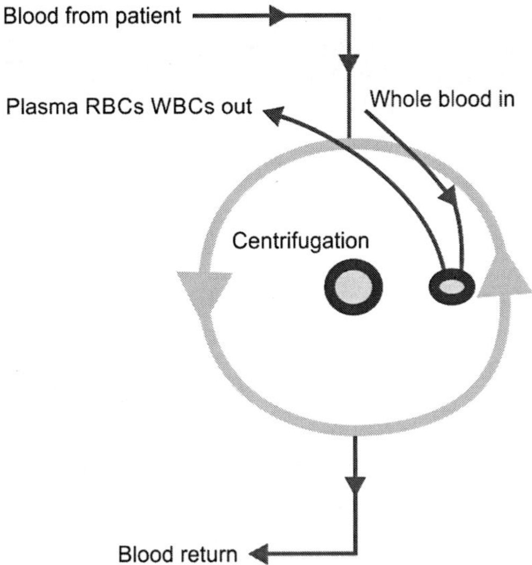

Fig. 1: Centrifugation plasma exchange.

Table 1: Intermittent vs continuous apheresis	
Intermittent TPE	***Continuous TPE***
Single sequential cycles	Continuous cycles
Two peripheral cannula or central venous catheter	Single peripheral cannula
Duration >4 hours	Lesser duration
Large extracorporeal volumes	Smaller volumes

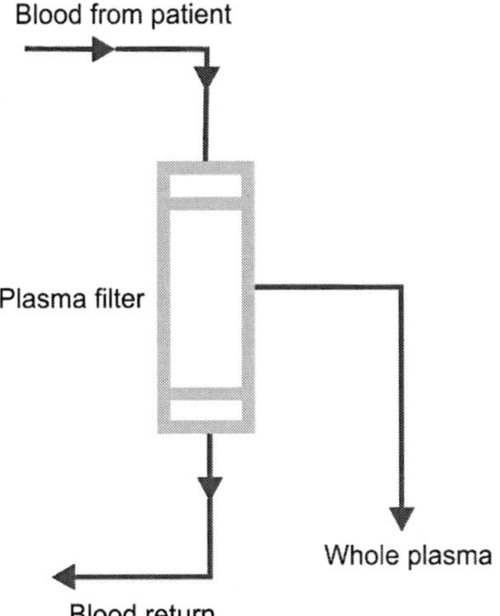

Fig. 2: Membrane plasma exchange.

is returned back to the patient. The procedure is usually performed using a hemodialysis machine.

Table 2 Comparison apheresis methods.

Table 2: Comparison apheresis methods.		
Features	Membrane TPE	Centrifugal TPE
Mechanism	Convection	Centrifugation
Anticoagulation	Heparin	Citrate
Blood flow, mL/min	100–250	10–150
Access	Central	Peripheral
Plasma extraction, %	30	80
Hyperviscosity syndrome	Reduced efficiency	Higher efficiency
Loss of platelets	Absent	Present
Separation	Molecular size	Specific gravity

Anticoagulation

- **Centrifugation:** Usually citrate is used in centrifugation plasma exchange. Infusion rate is according to blood flow rate 1:10 to 1:25. It also chelates calcium and can cause hypocalcemia.
- **Heparin:** It's usually used in membrane plasma exchange. Dose used is 40 U/kg followed by 20 U/kg/hr continuous infusion.

INDICATIONS FOR THERAPEUTIC PLASMA EXCHANGE

TPE is carried out in accordance with the American Society of Apheresis (AFSA) conditions as below.

Plasmapheresis for Neurologic Disorders

- Myasthenia gravis
- Multiple Sclerosis
- Acute inflammatory demyelinating polyneuropathy or Guillain-Barre syndrome
- Chronic inflammatory demyelinating neuropathy
- Polyneuropathy associated with IgA and IgG monoclonal gammopathy of undetermined significance (MGUS).

Plasmapheresis for Hematological Diseases

- Red cell alloimmunization in pregnancy
- Autoimmune hemolytic anemia
- Pure red cell aplasia
- Graft vs host disease
- ABO incompatible hematopoietic stem cell transplantation
- Cold agglutinin disease

Plasmapheresis for Autoimmune Diseases

- Severe SLE
- Lupus nephritis
- Catastrophic APLA

Plasmapheresis for Renal Disorders

- Antiglomerular basement membrane (anti-GBM) disease (good pasture syndrome)
- Crescentic rapidly progressive glomerulonephritis (not associated with anti-GBM antibody)
- Renal failure in multiple myeloma
- IgA nephropathy and Henoch-Schönlein purpura
- Thrombotic thrombocytopenic purpura
- Hemolytic uremic syndrome
- Scleroderma
- Focal segmental glomerulosclerosis: Recurrence post-transplantation
- Renal allograft rejection
- Renal transplantation across blood group type ABO groups

Complications (Table 3)

Table 3: Complications.

Feature	*Complications*
Vascular access	• Hematomas • Catheter-related infections • Thrombosis
Replacement fluid-related	• Viral infection transmission • Hypocalcemia • Hypokalemia • Coagulopathies • Anaphylaxis
Others	• Thrombocytopenia • Hypotension • ARDS • Arrhythmias • Myocardial Infarction

Replacement Fluids

- **5% Albumin:**
    - It's usually preferred replacement fluid in therapeutic plasma exchange
    - It's combined with normal saline in a ratio of 50:50 or 70:30
- **Saline:** It has low oncotic pressure. It's given usually in combination with other replacement fluids
- **Plasma:**
    - Plasma is usually preferred in TTP, liver disease and DIC
    - It's used as first line in thrombotic thrombocytopenic purpura
    - Physiological and maintains oncotic pressure
    - Provides proteins and clotting factors

Vascular Access

In TPE usually a central venous access is required especially when multiple exchanges are planned. In postrenal transplant patients AVF or graft is ideal for various indications. Care of the vascular access is equally important including prevention of catheter-related infections and sepsis.

Other Techniques

- **Cascade/double filtration:** Its re-filtration through secondary filter of smaller pore size. It removes larger unwanted molecules.
- **Cryofiltration:** It cools the plasma causing certain substances to aggregate (cryoglobulins, immune complexes).
- **Immunoadsorption:** Its nonselective removal of immunoglobulins and LDL cholesterol.
- **Hemadsorption**: It's used for the treatment of sepsis, removal of endotoxins and bacterial toxins.

SUGGESTED READING

1. Cervantes CE, Bloch EM, Sperati CJ. Therapeutic Plasma Exchange: Core Curriculum 2023. Am J Kidney Dis. 2023;81(4):475-92.
2. Clark WF, Huang SS. Introduction to therapeutic plasma exchange. Transfus Apher Sci. 2019;58(3):228-29.
3. Fernández-Zarzoso M, Gómez-Seguí I, de la Rubia J. Therapeutic plasma exchange: Review of current indications. Transfus Apher Sci. 2019;58(3):247-53.

Extracorporeal Therapies and Hemoperfusion

Kamal Sud, Sachin Srivastava, Narinder Pal Singh

INTRODUCTION

Extracorporeal therapies, also known as extracorporeal treatments (ECTR), are medical procedures that involve removing blood from the body, treating it outside the body, and then returning it to the patient. Various mechanisms involved in ECTRs for management of poisoning are, solute adsorption in hemoperfusion, diffusion in conventional hemodialysis (HD), convection as in hemofiltration or their combination as in hemodiafiltration (HDF), plasmapheresis for mushroom poisoning and drug overdose.

Continuous Kidney Replacement Therapy (CKRT), Sustained Low-efficiency Dialysis (SLED)

CKRT is a form of extracorporeal therapy used in hemodynamically unstable patients who are unable to tolerate the hemodynamic changes associated with conventional hemodialysis. SLED is a hybrid modality that is typically administered as a protracted therapy utilizing slower blood and dialysate flow rates.

Therapeutic Apheresis

Therapeutic apheresis encompasses various procedures that selectively remove certain components from the blood, such as specific antibodies, toxins, or abnormal cells. These procedures include plasmapheresis, cytapheresis (removal of specific cell types), and immunoadsorption (removal of specific antibodies).

In plasmapheresis, plasma is separated from the blood cells and is used in the management of some poisonings. The recommended exchange volume is equivalent to one to two total plasma volumes per day to treat there poisonings.

HEMOPERFUSION

Hemoperfusion, also known as **hemadsorption** is an extracorporeal blood purification procedure that involves the removal of toxins and other harmful substances (e.g., cytokines) from the blood using a specialized filter ('Column') containing adsorbent particles.

Principles of Hemoperfusion

Hemoperfusion operates on the principle of adsorption. Sorbent particles have characteristic large surface area to volume ratio. Physical adsorption works to bind substances and is controlled by factors such as molecule size, lipophilicity, hydrophobic interactions, van der waals interactions, hydrogen bonds, and ionic attraction. The hemoperfusion cartridge (or column) has adsorbent particles comprising activated charcoal or resins, which include hydrocarbon polymer, polystyrene. Charcoal has a stronger attraction for water-soluble molecules, while resins have greater binding for lipid-soluble molecules.

Indications for Hemoperfusion

Hemoperfusion is utilized in the management of various conditions involving the accumulation of toxic substances in the blood. The elimination of toxins that are lipid-soluble and highly protein-bound, such as in cases of poisoning, are poorly removed with conventional hemodialysis. Additionally, the elimination of cytokines in sepsis, the eradication of endotoxins or pathogens, the elimination of antibodies in autoimmune disorders, and the elimination of hepatic toxins in cases of liver failure are other potential applications of this procedure.

Overdose and Poisoning

It is particularly useful in cases of drug overdose, such as those involving salicylates, barbiturates, theophylline, methotrexate, carbamazepine, amanita mushrooms and certain toxins like **paraquat, if performed within few hours of ingestion.**

Acute Intoxications

Hemoperfusion is also employed in acute intoxications caused by substances such as methanol, ethylene glycol, or certain heavy metals like lead, mercury, or arsenic.

The following **Table 1** enlists common drugs and toxins that can be removed with Hemoperfusion.

Hemoperfusion Procedure

The hemoperfusion procedure involves several key steps:

Vascular Access

A large-bore central venous catheter is inserted into a major vein, usually the femoral or internal jugular vein.

Hemoperfusion Cartridge Setup

The hemoperfusion cartridge **(Fig. 1)** containing the adsorbent material, is connected to the extracorporeal circuit. The blood flow is directed through the cartridge, allowing toxins to be adsorbed onto the adsorbent surface.

Hemoperfusion Process

Blood is circulated by a pump through a sorbent unit (cartridge or column) and comes in direct contact with the sorbent particles **(Fig. 2)**.

Table 1: Common drugs and toxins removed with Hemoperfusion.

Acetylsalicylic acid	Phenytoin	Pentamidine	Ifosfamide
Acetaminophen	Promethazine	Methotrexate	Doxorubicin
Amitriptyline	Phenylbutazone	Isoniazid	Endosulfan
Chlorpromazine	Phenobarbital	Salicylic acid	Paraquat
Chloroquine	Valproic acid	Chloramphenicol	Parathion
Carbamazepine	Vancomycin	Dapsone	Amanitin
Colchicine	Chloral hydrate	Thiopental	Methyl parathion

(Adapted from: Blake BT, Ing TS. Handbook of dialysis/[edited by] John T. Daugirdas, Peter G. Blake, Todd S. 5th Ed, Wolters Kluwer Health; 2015)

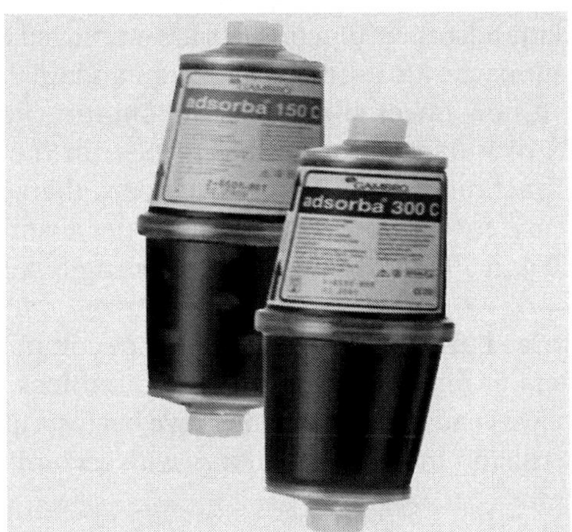

Fig. 1: Adsorba cartridge by Baxter (cellulose coated activated carbon).

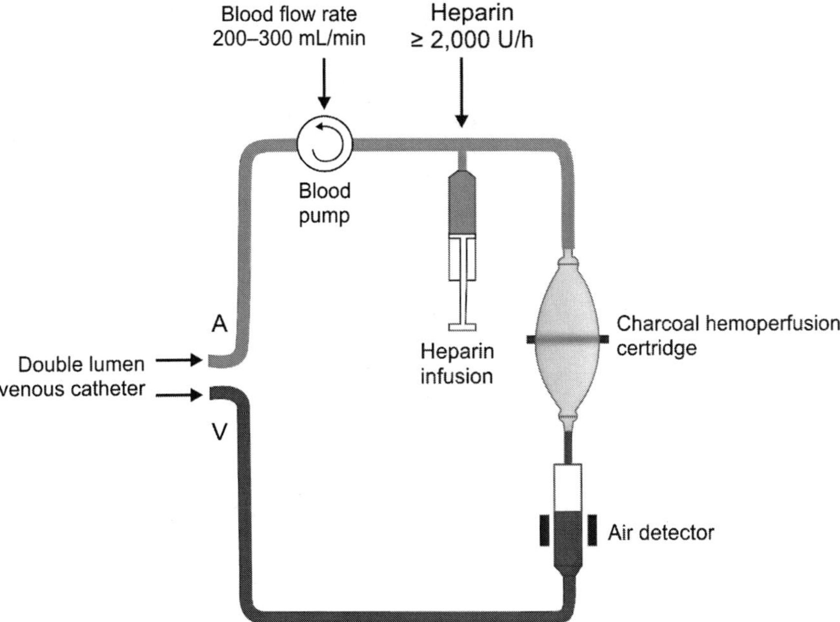

Fig. 2: Extracorporeal circuit for hemoperfusion.

(*Source:* Comprehensive clinical nephrology, 7th edition by Elsevier publication).

Complications

Thrombocytopenia, is the main adverse effect associated with hemoperfusion. It generally resolves within 1–2 days postprocedure. In addition, patients can experience hypotension, hypocalcemia, and hypoglycemia.

EXTRACORPOREAL THERAPY IN SEPSIS

Utilizing hemoperfusion with cartridges containing sorbents, researchers have attempted to manage sepsis by inactivating or removing endotoxin and/or inflammatory cytokines. This helps to attenuate the systemic inflammatory response associated with sepsis and may improve patient outcomes.

CytoSorb® (Fig. 3) is a cytokine adsorber (Biocon Ltd). It is employed in patients with sepsis with ongoing systemic inflammation who are not responding to standard therapy. It is recommended to be used in patients with new onset shock within 24 hours, increasing requirement of vasopressors, rising levels of inflammatory markers (Serum IL6 and Procalcitonin) and development of organ dysfunction even on optimal standard therapy. Continuous therapy is preferred over intermittent use, for a maximum of 24 hours per adsorbent cartridge. Blood flow rate should be between 150 and 500 mL/min. CytoSorb set-up before hemodialyser is shown in **Figure 4**.

Toraymyxin (Toray Industries Ltd) is hemoperfusion device composed of polymyxin B bound to polystyrene derived fibers. It binds to endotoxins and reduces plasma IL6 Levels and is indicated in patients with sepsis caused by gram-negative bacteria along with features of SIRS. It is used as direct hemoperfusion therapy for 2 hours with recommended blood flow rate of 80–120 mL/min.

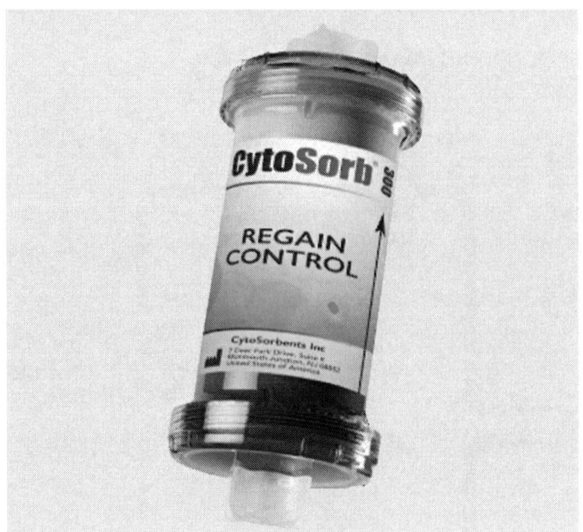

Fig. 3: CytoSorb® Extracorporeal cytokine adsorber by Biocon.

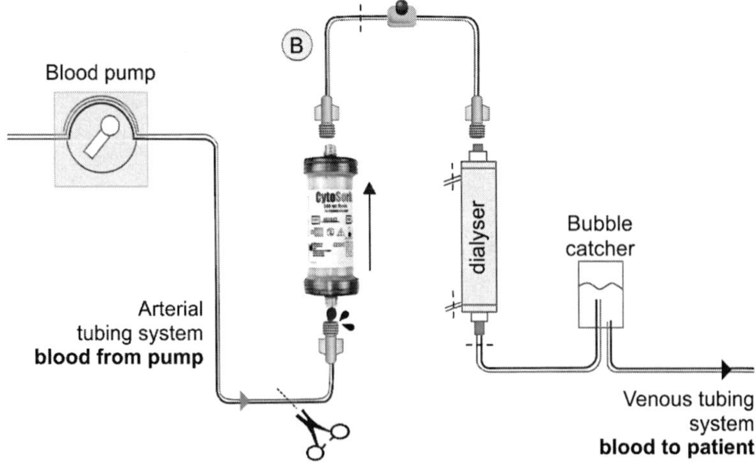

Fig. 4: Circuit diagram—CytoSorb set up before hemodialyser.

Extracorporeal Therapy in ABO Incompatible Transplants

It is used as part of desensitization protocol in ABO incompatible kidney transplant to remove antibodies. Plasma is passed through the immunoadsorption "column" at max flow rate of 50 mL/min and then reinfused back into the patient. ABO Adsopak® columns (POCARD Ltd, Moscow, Russia) **(Fig. 5)** and Glycosorb® ABO column (Glycorex Transplantation AB, Lund, Sweden) can be used. Glycosorb is a low-molecular-weight carbohydrate column with A or B blood group antigen **(Fig. 6)**. In the recipient, the Glycosorb-A column depletes anti-A antibody and the Glycosorb-B column depletes anti-B antibody.

Dialysis in Myeloma

The most prevalent cause of renal failure in multiple myeloma patients is light chain cast nephropathy. Due to the precipitation of light chains, the formation of casts causes tubular obstruction. In addition to chemotherapy, high cut-off dialysis and plasma exchange have been explored to remove these light chains. In myeloma patients with renal failure, hemodialysis using "High Cut-off" dialysers with a pore size of 50 kDa has been attempted with some favorable results in prevalents with k-free light chain myeloma.

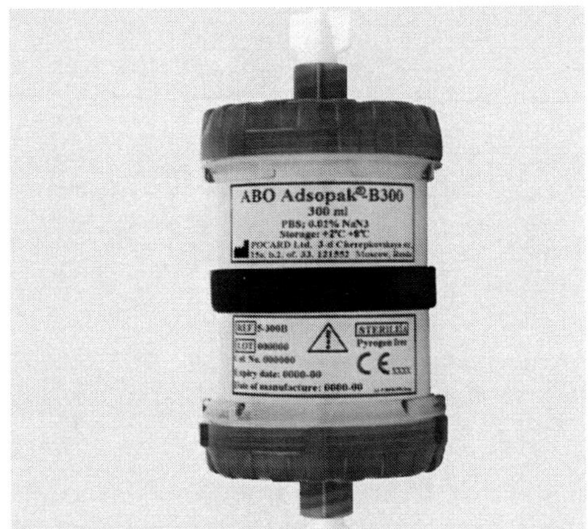

Fig. 5: ABO Adsopak® columns (POCARD Ltd, Moscow, Russia).

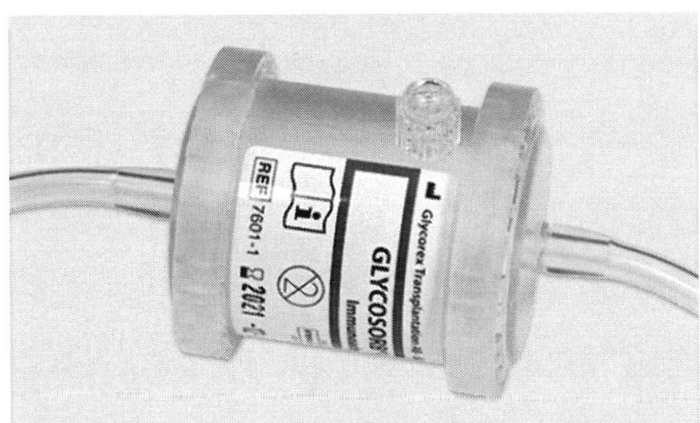

Fig. 6: Glycosorb® ABO column (Glycorex Transplantation AB, Lund, Sweden).

SUGGESTED READING

1. Ronco C, Bellomo R. Hemoperfusion: Technical aspects and state of the art. Crit Care. 2022;26(1):135. doi: 10.1186/s13054-022-04009-w. PMID: 35549999
2. Stegmayr B, Ramlow W, Balogun RA. Beyond dialysis: Current and emerging blood purification techniques. Semin Dial. 2012;25(2):207-13. doi: 10.1111/j.1525-139X.2011.01034.x. PMID: 22428812.
3. Clark WR, Ferrari F, La Manna G, Ronco C. Extracorporeal sorbent technologies: Basic concepts and clinical application. Contrib Nephrol. 2017;190:43-57. doi: 10.1159/000468911. Epub 2017 May 23. PMID: 28535518.
4. Mukherjee D, Hooda AK, Jairam A, Nair RK, Sharma S. Use of immunoadsorption columns in ABO-incompatible renal transplantation: A prospective study at a tertiary care center in India. Med J Armed Forces India. 2021;77(1):15-21. doi: 10.1016/j.mjafi.2019.08.005

Hemodialysis in Special Situations

Sachin Srivastava, Divya Bajpai, Arpita Roy Chowdhury

INTRODUCTION

Conventional hemodialysis procedure requires a good functioning vascular access, from which blood is passed through a "optimal sized" dialyser which effectively removes toxins and then blood if pumped back to patient. This process requires good understanding of patient's hemodynamic status, pathological state, type of vascular access, dialysis equipment and goals of dialysis therapy. In this chapter we will discuss practical considerations when hemodialysis is required in these special conditions.

DIALYSIS IN CRITICALLY ILL

Dialysis is challenging for critically ill patients. Due to their increased risk of hypotension, bleeding, infection, and other comorbidities, they are not suitable candidates for conventional HD. Sustained low efficiency dialysis (SLED) is a convenient option can be given with standard HD machines. As compared to "standard hemodialysis," it has lower blood flow rates and can be extended to 8–10 hours in order to achieve greater urea "clearance." For example, (dialysis prescription for SLED: Duration- 6–8 hrs, blood flow of 150–250 mL/min, dialysate flow of 200–300 mL/min, Anticoagulation: UFH or saline, and access-AVF/catheter). It can be administered at night, allowing patients to undergo diagnostic and interventional procedures during the day. Continuous renal replacement therapy (CRRT) is another modality for dialysis in the critically ailing. Continuous dialysis is carried out at a much slower rate (blood flow 100–200 mL/min) and for a longer duration (usually 48–72 hours). Few limitations of CRRT include a higher cost per treatment, the need for sophisticated equipment, and the need for technical expertise.

DIALYSIS IN PREGNANCY

Management of a pregnant patient of dialysis is tough. Recommendations are for initiation of dialysis once glomerular filtration rate is less than 20 mL/min or blood urea nitrogen (BUN) >100 mg/dL. The frequency of hemodialysis sessions is at least 5 days/week or min 20 hrs/week. A practical target is maintaining blood urea nitrogen (BUN) levels less than 50 mg/dL. The recommended potassium levels in the dialysate between 3.0 and 3.5 mmol/L. It is advisable to administer lower doses of bicarbonate in the dialysate, specifically at 25 mmol/L (instead of 28–32 mmol/L), due to the potential elevation of metabolic alkalosis risk associated with frequent hemodialysis. Maintenance of stable hemodynamic status and avoidance of hypotension is very important. Patients, after delivery can go back to previous prepregnancy dialysis schedule.

DIALYSIS IN ELDERLY

Initiation and maintenance of hemodialysis in elderly patients need certain special considerations. In general, most elderly patients have limited body reserves, likely to have more comorbidities, higher complication rate from dialysis, vascular access issues, symptoms of frailty, and higher susceptibility for infections.

There is likelihood of delayed maturation of AVF as compared to younger patients. Several factors have been identified as independent predictors of poor survival, including advanced age (85 years or older), poor nutritional and functional status, cognitive impairment, dependence on assistance for daily activities, delayed referral for dialysis initiation, initiation of dialysis during hospitalization, the presence of other comorbidities, particularly involving cardiovascular and central nervous system. There doesn't seem to be a simple way to treat ESRD in older people, but patient-centered, goal-directed therapy, which is based on shared decision-making between the doctor and the patient, should make it easier to choose a dialysis schedule that will relieve symptoms while reducing the adverse effects of treatment.

DIALYSIS IN CHILDREN

It is demanding to care for pediatric patients who require renal replacement treatment. Indications for urgent initiation of dialysis in pediatric patients is generally same as those of adults (refractory hyperkalemia, severe metabolic acidosis, refractory volume overload, uremic encephalopathy, and uremic pericarditis). A good arteriovenous fistula for maintenance dialysis is possible in children more than 9 years. As a result, in infants and children, peritoneal dialysis is the recommended modality. In infants, the PD exchange volume is 30–50 mL/kg.

Hemodialysis Equipment in Children

Table 1 shows size of catheters and dialysers used in pediatric patients.

Anticoagulation: Initial loading dose of 20 U/kg of unfractionated heparin is given followed by continuous infusion of 10 U/Kg/hr.

Blood flow rates: For initial dialysis session, it is advisable not to exceed blood flow rates more than 4–5 mL/kg/min, which can be gradually increased to 8 mL/Kg/min in subsequent HD sessions.

Dialysate flow rates: In patients weighing less than 20 kgs, dialysate flow rate must be maintained between 300 and 500 mL/min. For children weighing more than 20 kgs, the dialysate flow rate can be kept at 500–800 mL/min.

Ultrafiltration rate is kept initially at 8 mL/Kg per hour and gradually escalated as per patients' tolerance to 10–12 mL/kg per hour. Ultrafiltration should not be greater than 5% of total body weight.

DIALYSIS IN POSTOPERATIVE PATIENT

Dialysis in a postoperative patient has certain important considerations. Immediate dialysis indications can be due to hyperkalemia or volume overload situations arising due to "stress" of surgery, blood transfusions or anesthetic drugs. Assessment of blood pressure and volume status in post of period is critical and will affect dialysis prescription. Close coordination with primary surgery and anesthesia team for discussion on vital issues like nature of surgical procedure,

Table 1: Showing size of catheters and dialysers used in pediatric patients wrt weight.

Patient age/Wt	*Vascular access size*	*Dialyser size*
Neonate	4–6 F single lumen catheter	F4 (0.8 sqm) or F5 (1.0 sqm)
3–6 kg	7 F double lumen catheter	
6–15 kg	8 F double lumen catheter	
15–30 kg	9 F double lumen catheter	
>30 kg	10 F double lumen catheter	F6 (1.3 sqm)

any unexpected complications during surgery, need of blood or components transfusion, parenteral nutrition, dose adjustment for antibiotics, plan for extubating and bleeding risk on anticoagulation. It is advisable to avoid or minimize anticoagulation with careful ultrafiltration for initial HD sessions in post op period when the risk is maximum.

Extracorporeal Membrane Oxygenation

Extracorporeal membrane oxygenation (ECMO) is a technique that provides both cardiac and respiratory support to patients with severe heart or lung failure. It involves pumping blood out of the body, oxygenating it using a membrane oxygenator, and then returning it to the patient's circulatory system. ECMO is beneficial for treating cardiac failure in individuals who are unable to wean from cardiopulmonary bypass or who cannot be treated with a ventricular assist device. ECMO should be considered in cases of potentially reversible but life-threatening respiratory failure. In cases of irreversible cardiac failure, ECMO resuscitation can serve as a bridge to heart transplantation or ventricular assist device.

Nocturnal Hemodialysis

HD session is given during night time at the dialysis center, while the patients is asleep. It has the advantage of an extended dialysis duration of 6–8 hours per session. It is performed three times a week. Nocturnal home hemodialysis, where HD therapy is given during night hours at home rather than incentre. It is more convenient for patients, who have a busy daytime schedule and prefer to avoid HD sessions during the day.

SUGGESTED READING

1. Corbett RW, Brown EA. Conventional dialysis in the elderly: How lenient should our guidelines be? Semin Dial. 2018;31:607-11. https://doi.org/10.1111/sdi.12744
2. Oliverio AL, Hladunewich MA. End-Stage Kidney Disease and Dialysis in Pregnancy. Adv Chronic Kidney Dis. 2020;27(6):477-85. doi: 10.1053/j.ackd.2020.06.001.
3. Wiles K, de Oliveira L. Dialysis in pregnancy. Best Pract Res Clin Obstet Gynaecol. 2019;57:33-46. doi: 10.1016/j.bpobgyn.2018.11.007. Epub 2018 Nov 27.

Procedures in Nephrology

Vineet Behera, Indradip Maity, AK Bhalla

INTRODUCTION

It is very crucial for dialysis technicians and nurses to know the basics about procedures in nephrology. They are needed to assist and help nephrologists in carrying out the procedures. The various procedures in nephrology one should know about are insertion of temporary hemodialysis catheters, tunneled cuffed catheters and kidney biopsy. Another procedure is CAPD catheter insertion, the scope of which is beyond this chapter.

List of Interventions in Nephrology

- Temporary hemodialysis catheter insertion
- Tunneled cuffed catheter (TCC) insertion
- TCC complication intervention—Disruption fibrin sheath, exchange TCC
- TCC removal
- Kidney biopsy
- PD catheter insertion
- PD catheter—other interventions (exchange, repositioning)
- PD catheter extrusion
- AV fistula creation
- AV fistula repair (psuedoaneurysm, thrombus)
- AV fistula baloon venoplasty
- Central vein endovascular interventions
- Renal artery interventions

INSERTION OF TEMPORARY HEMODIALYSIS CATHETERS (JUGULAR, FEMORAL, SUBCLAVIAN)

For successful dialysis it is very important to secure vascular access into a major vein. Seldinger method is used for the same and nowadays USG guided cannulation is done in places where it is available. Jugular vein is preferred (internal > external), followed by femoral and then subclavian. The right jugular vein is preferred as it drains directly into the superior vena cava and right atrium.

Items Needed for Cannulation

- Sterile tray with small bowls, cotton balls, gauze pieces, sponge holding forceps, and needle holder.
- 5 mL Syringe with needle for local anesthesia administration.
- Sterile pack of new catheter kit with catheter, guidewire, dilators, introducer needle—(catheter kit contains all these), one must ensure that the length of catheter is chosen adequately, generally 14.5 French, 11 cm catheter is used for right jugular temporary access.
- Betadine, adhesive plaster

For cannulating internal jugular vein, patient should lie over a small sandbag in the upper part of the chest. Neck should be turned to the opposite side. The internal jugular vein is identified by the following way. The sternocleidomastoid muscle extends from mastoid process till sternum and clavicle on each side where it gets inserted as two heads. The apex where the two heads separate is the landmark. When USG was not available, the pulsation of the internal carotid artery was identified and just lateral to it, skin is anesthetized with lignocaine after cleaning the area with betadine. A 18–20 g needle is used to locate the vein and is directed at 45 degrees in the direction of nipple. The needle is introduced with slow aspiration till dark red blood is aspirated, after this the introducer needle is inserted close to the guiding needle. After venous blood is aspirated, J tip guidewire is introduced in the vein. The needle is removed and then serial dilators are introduced. First, the dilation by small dilator is followed by dilation by larger dilator in a rotating fashion, always ensuring the movement of the guidewire back and forth is smooth. After dilating the tract, catheter is introduced over the guidewire, and the guidewire is removed after securing the catheter. Catheter lumens are flushed with normal saline after checking flow, and then ports are locked with heparinized saline. A chest X-ray is done to check position of catheter tip. The catheter tip should be in the junction of SVC and RA, once catheter position is confirmed, hemodialysis is initiated. In real time USG guidance, the jugular vein is punctured under real time guidance, the guidewire course into the SVC can be tracked via USG and then the steps are the same.

For femoral cannulation **(Fig. 1)**, femoral artery is palpated in the upper thigh, approximately 1 inch below the middle of inguinal ligament, the vein is located medial to the artery and after puncturing the vein the steps are same as above. Subclavian cannulation should be used as a last resort as there is high chance of subclavian vein stenosis. The landmark is below the collar bone, approximately between middle and outer third of the collar bone. The needle is directed below, then parallel to the bed pointing towards opposite sternoclavicular joint. As the needle tip enters the subclavian vein blood enters the syringe and the next steps are same as that of jugular vein cannulation.

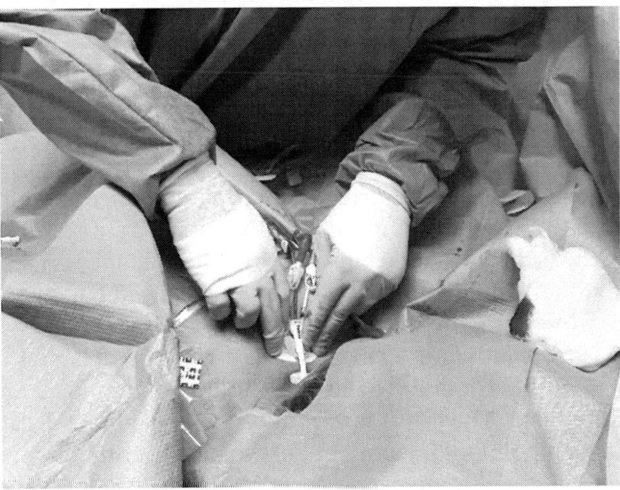

Fig. 1: Femoral cannulation for dialysis catheter.

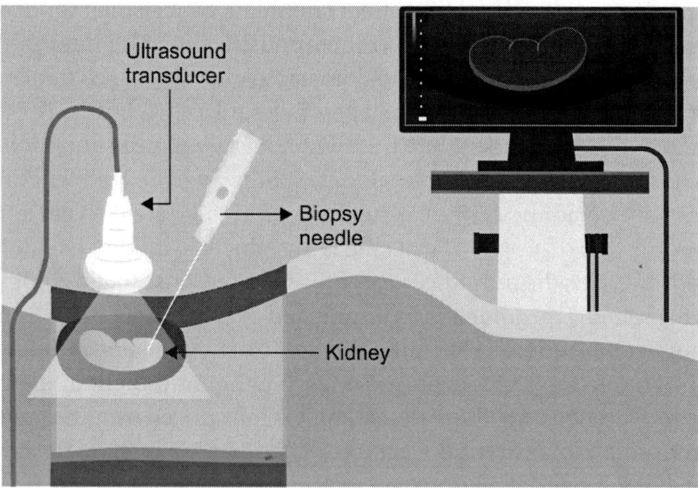

Fig. 2: Diagrammatic representation of kidney biopsy.

KIDNEY BIOPSY (FIG. 2)

Left kidney is generally preferred for biopsy. Patient is placed in prone position and a sandbag/ pillow is placed under the abdomen. Under USG guidance the lower pole of kidney is identified. The area is thoroughly cleaned with betadine solution, then cut sheet is applied. Under real time USG guidance, local anesthesia is given with 2% lignocaine under USG guidance. After anesthesia, spring loaded kidney biopsy gun 16 g × 16 cm or 18 g × 16 cm is inserted along the same tract under USG guidance. The gun is inserted till ½ cm from the renal capsule of the lower pole of the kidney. Patient is asked to hold breath and then the gun is fired. The biopsy core is taken and transferred into formalin, normal saline and glutaraldehyde vials. Generally, 2–3 cores are taken. After the procedure, kidney is screened by USG for any hematoma or bleeding. Local pressure is generally applied for 10–15 minutes, after this the patient is turned and made to lie flat for the next 12 hours, and the urine is monitored for any hematuria. The complications of kidney biopsy include perinephric hematoma, hematuria, AV aneurysm formation in kidney, intra-abdominal bleed, infection, bladder clots, and others.

TUNNELED CUFFED DIALYSIS CATHETER (TCC) INSERTION (FIG. 3)

TCC should always be inserted under C Arm fluoroscopic guidance and ultrasound guidance. For right jugular vein, a 19 cm sized TCC is used. The initial steps are same as temporary dialysis catheter access. After inserting the guidewire, fluoroscopic guidance is used to ensure that the guidewire in placed into the inferior vena cava. Thereafter, a subcutaneous tunnel is created using the trocar ensuring a smooth curve of the catheter. Subcutaneous tunnel is generally created around 2 finger breadth (1.5–2 cm) below the junction of lateral 1/3 and medial 2/3 of clavicle which acts as the exit site. The area is infiltrated with local anesthesia from exit site to needle puncture point. The trocar is introduced after loading the catheter and inserted subcutaneously from exit point till it comes out of the needle entry point. Sometimes a small incision of skin might be given in the needle insertion to facilitate easy passage of the trocar. The cuff of the TCC should be inside the tunnel about 2–3 cm from the exit point. Then serial dilators are used over the guidewire under fluoro guidance to dilate the tract. The peel away sheath is introduced over the guidewire, the guidewire is removed and then the catheter is introduced through the sheath. After the catheter has passed halfway the peel away sheath is

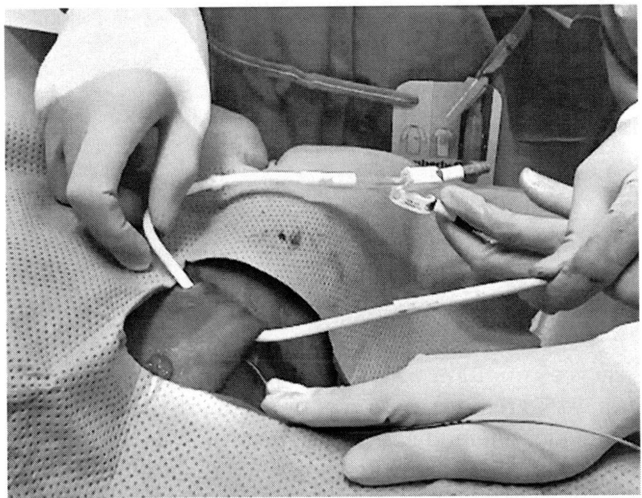

Fig. 3: Tunneled cuffed dialysis catheter (TCC) insertion.

broken and the catheter is slowly introduced while peeling away the sheath. The final position of catheter tip should be at the RA-SVC junction. The flow of both lumens are checked and locked with heparin. The incision points are sutured and anchor sutures are applied over the TCC. Appropriate dressing is done.

SUGGESTED READING

1. Efstratiadis G, Platsas I, Koukoudis P, Vergoulas G. Interventional nephrology: A new subspecialty of nephrology. Hippokratia. 2007;11(1):22-4.
2. Niyyar VD, Beathard G. Interventional Nephrology: Opportunities and Challenges. Adv Chronic Kidney Dis. 2020;27(4):344-349.e1.
3. Yevzlin AS, Asif A, Salman L, Ramani K, Qaqish SS, Vachharajani TJ. Interventional Nephrology. Springer International Publishing; 2022.

Peritoneal Dialysis

26
CHAPTER

Pavitra Manu Dogra, Vineet Behera, Ranjith Kumar Nair

INTRODUCTION

Chronic kidney disease is a condition where the body's waste products are retained due to poorly functioning kidneys. To remove these accumulated waste products, renal replacement therapy is given, which includes hemodialysis, peritoneal dialysis, and kidney transplantation. Peritoneal dialysis (PD) is one of the many forms of renal replacement therapies available for managing advanced chronic kidney disease, acute kidney disease, and chronic fluid overload due to chronic congestive cardiac failure. This method utilizes the semipermeable property of the human peritoneum. It is a very good modality of dialysis wherein the patient enjoys freedom from mandatory hospital visits for rigid and fixed dialysis slots for in-hospital hemodialysis. This freedom offered by peritoneal dialysis allows the patients to undertake travels, and continue with their profession and jobs, thereby leading a satisfied life with good quality.

TYPES OF PERITONEAL DIALYSIS

PD procedure consists of infusing dialysate fluid into the peritoneal cavity, dwelling it for a limited time to allow exchanges of electrolytes and waste products, and then removal of the effluent from the peritoneal cavity. This is usually done with the help of a PD catheter, usually made of silicon. The various types of PD are as follows:

1. **Acute peritoneal dialysis (Acute PD):** This is the type of peritoneal dialysis that is done for acute kidney injury. An acute PD catheter, either rigid or soft PD catheter is used. The usual period of use is 24–72 hours. Initial cycles are time-bound Thereafter the rigid PD catheter is either removed or replaced by a soft silicon PD catheter for continuing PD beyond 72 hours.
2. **Continuous ambulatory peritoneal dialysis (CAPD):** CAPD consists of 3–4 exchanges per day, with either night dwell or night dry **(Fig. 1)**. The day exchanges are usually 4 hours each and the night exchange is prolonged to 10–12 hours.
3. **Automated peritoneal dialysis (APD):** This is a form of PD in which exchanges are done by a machine **(Fig. 2)**. Ten liters of PD fluid is exchanged by the machine overnight. This may be followed by a long day dwell of a hypertonic solution, commonly used as 2 liters of 7.5% icodextrin solution. This is of many types depending on the kind of exchange schedule used. The commoner ones are continuous cyclical PD (CCPD), in which 2 hourly exchanges are done overnight, followed by a day dwell of 2 liters of 7.5% icodextrin solution, and night intermittent PD (NIPD) in which two hourly exchanges are done overnight without any day dwell.

PD CATHETERS

There are many types of PD catheters that have found their place in the history of PD in past seven decades. Few of these are Toronto Western, Missouri, disc catheters, and lead ball catheters. But today, the following PD catheters are being used.

1. **Acute PD catheter (Fig. 3).**

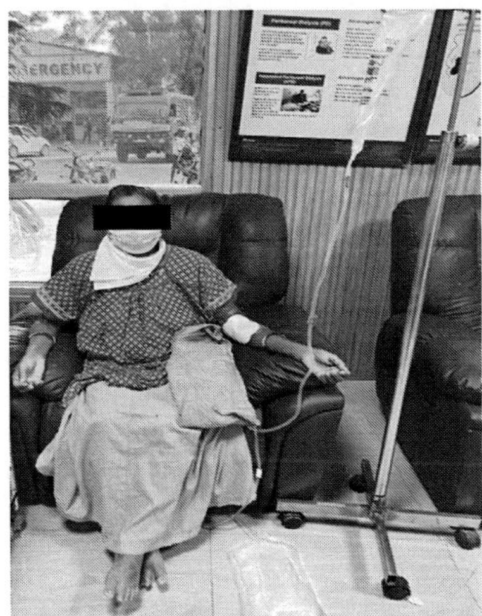

Fig. 1: Chronic ambulatory peritoneal dialysis.

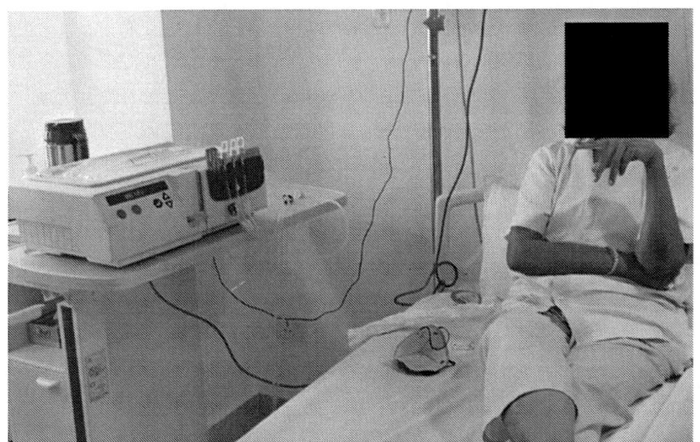

Fig. 2: Automated peritoneal dialysis.

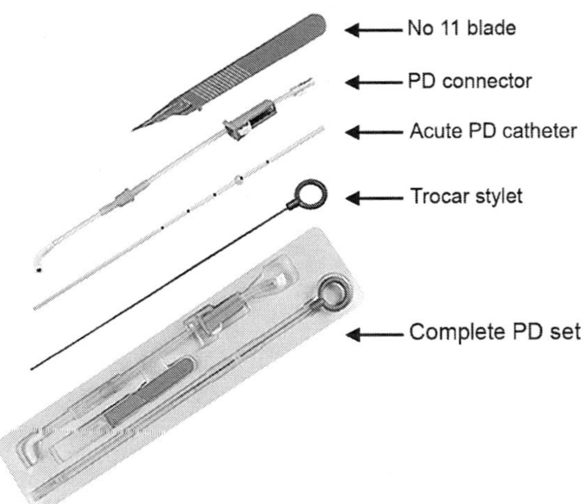

Fig. 3: Acute PD catheter.

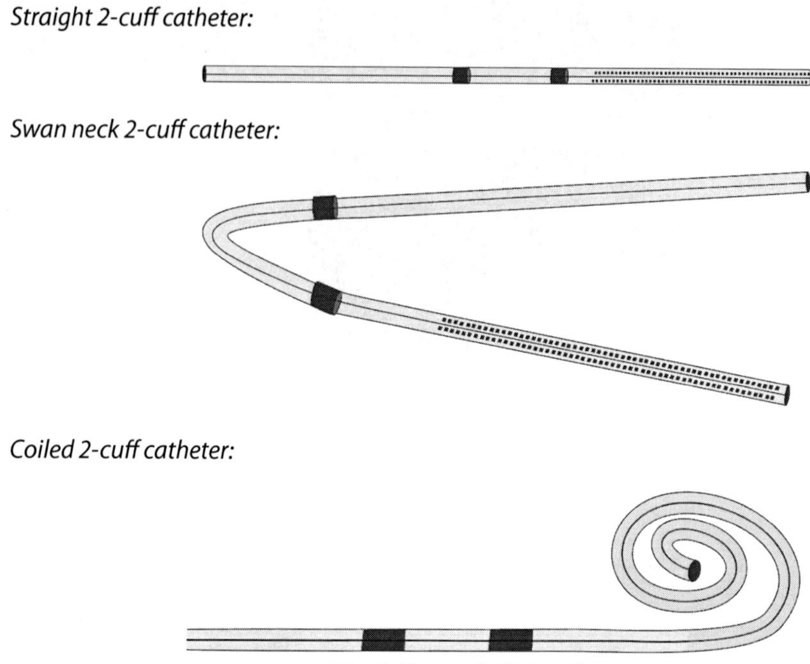

Fig. 4: Types of CAPD catheters.

2. **CAPD catheter:** There are three main types of CAPD catheters used now. They have multiple holes in the distal third of the catheter and two cuffs for fixing the PD catheter. Each PD catheter has a white radiopaque line placed anteriorly and centrally for easy visualization on the roentgenogram. These are given in **Figure 4**.

METHODS OF INSERTION

1. **Acute PD catheter insertion (percutaneous rigid catheter) (Fig. 5):** This is done in emergency situations. This is a rigid catheter inserted via a stab incision in the midline infraumbilical region.

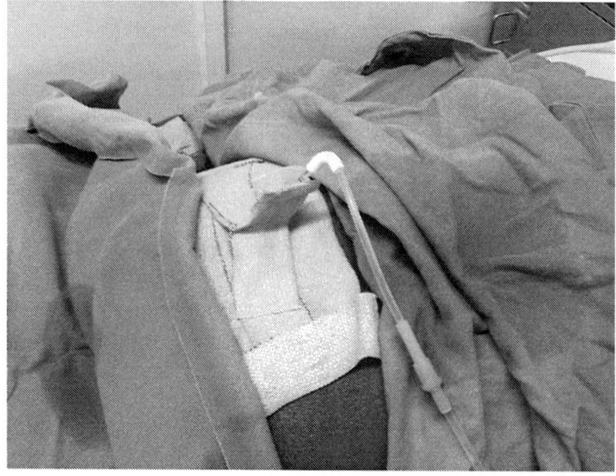

Fig. 5: Acute PD catheter insertion.

2. **CAPD catheter insertion:** This is done for long-term peritoneal dialysis. A two-cuffed silicon PDC is inserted by the following techniques.
   a. *Percutaneous insertion* **(Fig. 6)**: This is done using Seldinger's technique.

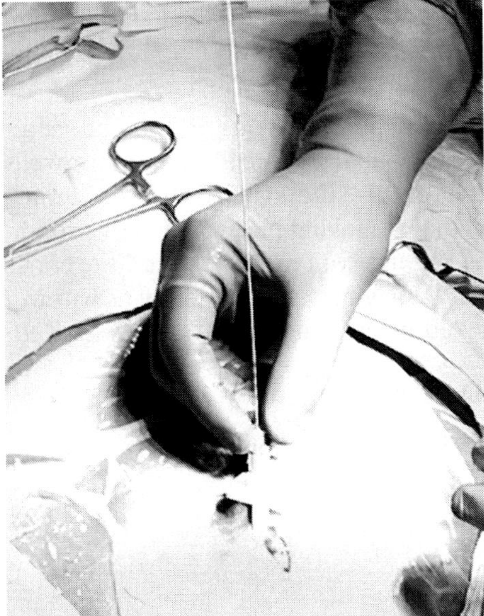

Fig. 6: Percutaneous CAPD catheter insertion.

   b. *Open dissection or laparoscopic insertion* **(Fig. 7)**: This is done via a paramedian incision by open dissection in which the PD catheter is placed through anterior rectus muscle belly. It can also be done laparoscopically.

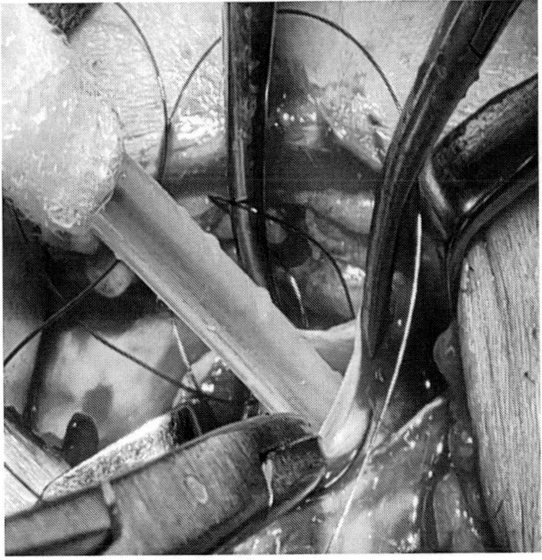

Fig. 7: Open CAPD catheter insertion.

Physiology of Peritoneal Dialysis

Peritoneal dialysis functions on principles of osmosis, diffusion, convection, and ultrafiltration. There are many models of PD. The two important ones which improve our understanding of exchanges through semi-permeable membrane. In the three-pore model, the molecules are exchanged across the membrane depending on the size of the pores. In the distributed model, the glucose concentration in PD fluid drives the filtration of fluid by osmosis thus causing osmotic ultrafiltration from the peritoneal capillaries to the peritoneal cavity.

CAPD PROCEDURE (FIG. 8)

Once a PD catheter is inserted by percutaneous or open dissection method, it is allowed to settle in for 10–14 days, whereas in laparoscopic PD insertion, dwells can be started in 3–5 days. Thereafter, three to four dwells of 1.5–3 liters (depending on surface area) for 3.5–4 hours each are initiated. The amount of dialysis taking place is directly proportional to the volume of the dwell, number of exchanges, regularity of exchanges and the concentration of dialysate fluid. In emergency situations, CAPD may be started as early as within 24 hours. This is known as urgent-start PD. In this low volume exchanges (500 mL) are started.

Contraindications to PD

- Multiple abdominal surgeries with adhesions
- Morbid obesity
- Unhealthy overlying skin
- Large abdominal aortic aneurysm
- ADPKD with large kidneys
- Recurrent inguinal hernia

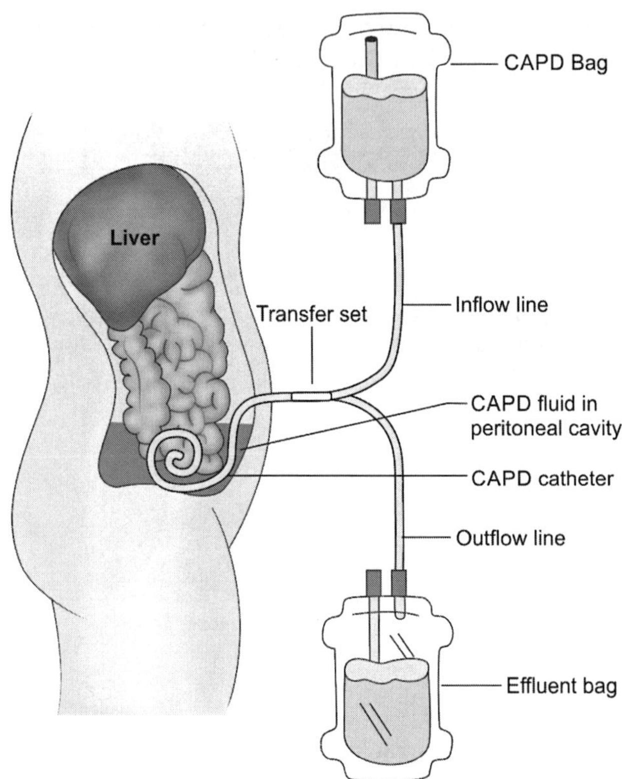

Fig. 8: Principle of CAPD exchange.

- Recurrent large umbilical hernia
- Patient with ostomies
- Altered mentation
- Patient with no social support and leading a solitary lifestyle
- Patient who is not convinced about this modality.

Complications of PD Catheter Insertion

- Bowel perforation
- Intra-abdominal vascular injury
- Preperitoneal placement of the catheter
- Urinary bladder injury
- Pericatheter dialysate leakage
- Incisional hernia
- Abdominal distension and breathing difficulty
- Hemorrhagic outflow
- Localized inflow and outflow pain

Late Complications of CAPD and APD

- PD peritonitis
- Ultrafiltration failure
- PD catheter migration
- PD catheter omental wrapping
- Hemorrhagic outflow
- Intestinal erosion by PD catheter
- Cuff extrusion
- Peritoneal-pleural communication leading to hydrothorax
- Fracture of PD catheter
- Chronic tunnel pain
- Incisional hernia

Role and Responsibilities of Dialysis Technician

- Understanding the functioning of the CAPD process.
- Assist in PD catheter insertion procedures.
- Counseling of patients for CAPD.
- Handling of CAPD complications to some extent.
- Become a bridge between the patient and the treating doctor.

SUGGESTED READING

1. Agarwal AK, Salman L, Asif A. Peritoneal Dialysis: Types, Procedures and Risks Factors (Renal and Urologic Disorders: Public Health in the 21st Century), 1st edition. Nova Biomedical.
2. Nolph and Gokal's Textbook of Peritoneal Dialysis, 3rd edition. Springer.
3. Rastogi A, Lerma EV, Bargman JM. Applied Peritoneal Dialysis Improving Patient Outcomes. Springer.

Renal Transplantation

27
CHAPTER

A Kishore Kumar, Subho Banerjee, Vivek Kute

INTRODUCTION

End-stage kidney disease (kidney failure) is a condition in which kidneys permanently cease to do their functions. If kidneys fail to do their job, all the waste products generated in the body accumulate, which can lead to death. To survive, the patient has to rely on dialysis or kidney transplantation. Kidney transplantation is a procedure in which a normal functioning kidney is taken from a living person or brain-dead patient and implanted into a patient suffering from kidney failure. Dialysis procedure can only replace 15% of kidney function. Whereas a new kidney via transplantation can do all the functions of a native kidney, improving patient well-being and longevity. The first successful kidney transplantation was done in 1954 by Dr Joseph Murray in 1954.

Kidney transplantation is the preferred treatment modality in kidney failure because:

- Patients who undergo transplantation live a longer life compared to those who remain on dialysis **(Fig. 1)**.
- Quality of life is better in patients with transplantation.
- The need for dialysis procedure is avoided improving the well-being of the patient.

Based on the source of the donor organ, a kidney transplant is classified as living donor transplantation or cadaveric (deceased-donor) transplantation.

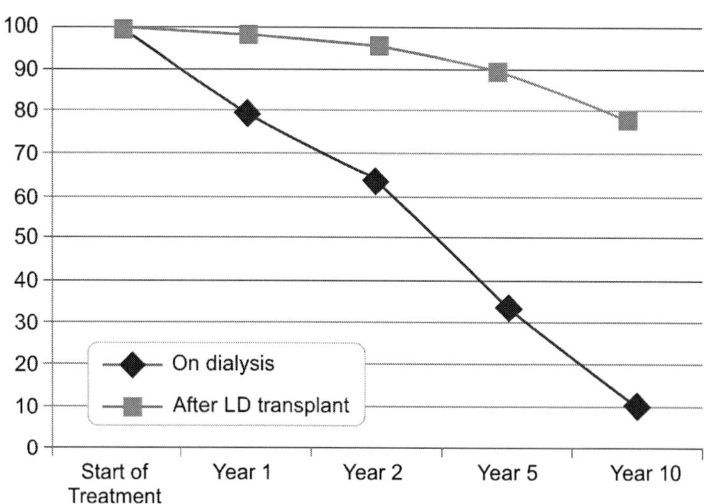

Fig. 1: Patients who undergo kidney transplantation live longer than those who remain on dialysis.
(*Source:* Continuing Education in Anaesthesia Critical Care and Pain Volume 12, Issue 6, December 2012, Pages 317-321)

TYPES KIDNEY TRANSPLANT

Living Donor Transplantation

Any living person willing to donate his kidney should be in a proper state of health and not be mentally challenged. He should be fit to donate the kidney.

Types of Living Donors

Living kidney donors can be any one of the following:
- Near-related donor (includes brother, sister, mother, father, son, daughter, grandmother, grandfather, grandson, and granddaughter)
- Spousal donor
- Donor other than a near relative

A donor other than a near relative can be a person who is a relative of the recipient (other than a near relative), neighbor, friend, etc., who is emotionally attached to the patient and want to donate without any monetary benefit.

Cadaveric (Deceased-donor) Transplantation

Deceased donors (cadaveric donors) are patients who are declared brain-dead by a team of experts. Organs from such donors are taken after the consent of immediate relatives for transplantation.

LIVING KIDNEY DONATION

- A living kidney donor is a person undergoing surgery to help the patient. The safety of the donor is paramount both during and after surgery over the long term.
- For a fit donor, kidney donation is usually uncomplicated and long-term outcomes are good. Risks of kidney donation are surgical risks like bleeding and postoperative infections.
- Over the long term, donors are at risk of developing hypertension, protein loss in the urine, and a mild increase in the risk of kidney disease. Young female donors are at risk of hypertension during pregnancy.
- Before donation donor undergoes a battery of tests to assess his kidney function and the general status of other organs in the body. Diabetic donors are usually excluded from donation. In the case of hypertension in the donor, if the blood pressure is controlled and there are no effects of hypertension on organs in the body, the donor is accepted.
- Before donation, hematological evaluation, thyroid evaluation, lipid profile, infection history and evaluation, liver function evaluation, chest X-ray, gynecological evaluation, and psychiatry evaluation are made. Regarding kidney function evaluation, tests like creatinine, urea, electrolytes, ultrasound abdomen, complete urine examination, and 24-hour urine albumin estimation are done. If these reports are within the normal range, then GFR is measured. The patient's fitness from specific specialist doctors is taken-based on the medical history of the patient.
- After the physical fitness of the donor, cross-matching between donor and recipient is done.
- For donors, laparoscopic donor nephrectomy is usually done, which is less invasive and recovery time is short. After donation, the donor is generally discharged in 3–5 days if there are no complications.
- After recovery, the donor can return to the previous routine. Blood pressure, kidney function and urine should be checked at three months and yearly after that.

Recipient Evaluation and Surgery

Before the transplantation, patients with kidney failure undergo extensive testing and evaluation.

- There are a few situations in which kidney transplantation is not advised, even if the patient has kidney failure. They include:
  - Active infection in the patient
  - Uncontrolled cancer
  - Drug addiction and dependence
  - Uncontrolled psychiatric illness
  - Short life expectancy of less than 1–2 years due to any condition
  - Positive cross-match (CDC) with donor
- Kidney failure patients should be adequately vaccinated before the transplantation to decrease the risk of infections. They are extensively tested for hematological parameters and liver, pulmonary, and cardiac function. Fitness from respective specialists is taken, and cross-matching with the donor is done. Based on the cross-match donor is accepted or rejected. If the cross-match report is positive, there is an increased risk of rejection after transplant-based on the type of cross-match.
- The native kidneys of the patient which failed are not removed. The new kidney from the donor is placed in the right iliac fossa, as shown in **Figure 2**. After the surgery, if everything goes well, there is brisk urine output and kidney function tests normalize gradually.
- The patient is started on medications to suppress his immunity and prevent rejection of the transplanted organ, which must continue lifelong.

RISKS OF KIDNEY TRANSPLANTATION

- After surgery, complications like bleeding, infections, and prolonged hospital stay.
- Immunosuppressive medications increase the risk of infections, a few types of cancers, and side effects specific to the drugs.
- There is a risk of organ rejection by the recipient's body at any time after transplant. Rejection risk increases if there is a positive cross-match and medications are not taken properly.

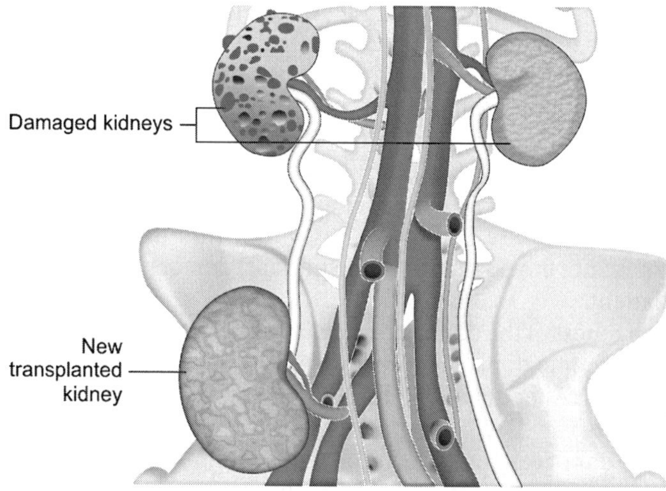

Fig. 2: New kidney is placed in the right iliac fossa, and damaged kidneys are not removed.

Rules and Regulations for Transplant in India

Kidney transplantation in India is done under the rules and regulations of the Govt. of India. These rules and regulations are mainly to avoid the illegal selling of organs for monetary benefit and to regulate the removal, storage, and transplantation of organs for treatment. The first act passed in 1994 was the Transplantation of Human Organs Act (THOA). Later the act was modified in 1995, 2008, 2011, and 2014. Ministry of Health and family welfare in 2014 notified the Transplantation of Human Organs and Tissue Rules, which is currently followed in the country.

SUGGESTED READING

1. Abramyan S, Hanlon M. Kidney Transplantation. [Updated 2023 Jan 2]. In: StatPearls [Internet]. Treasure Island (FL): StatPearls Publishing; 2024
2. Guidelines of Kidney Transplantation. NOTTO. Ministry of Health and family Welfare. Govt of India.
3. KDIGO Clinical Practice Guideline on the Evaluation and Management of Candidates for Kidney Transplantation. Transplantation. 2020;104(4S1):S11-S103.

Nutrition in Chronic Kidney Disease

Gaurav Batta, NK Medi, NK Mattewada, KS Nayak

INTRODUCTION

Malnutrition or protein energy wasting syndrome (PEW) is very common in patients on dialysis and can lead to impaired immune function, and in turn increased susceptibility to infections, more hospitalizations and premature death. It's seen in 50–70% of patients on dialysis and hence it's important to screen for malnutrition periodically.

Causes of Malnutrition

The common causes for poor nutrition are:
- Anorexia due to inadequate dialysis or retention of uremic toxins
- Intercurrent illnesses
- Chronic systemic inflammation
- Metabolic acidosis
- Depression

Assessment

There is no single measurement that can determine malnutrition hence it is best to use a combination of different valid measures mentioned below. Assessment is recommended to be done by a registered dietitian nutritionist (RDN) at periodic intervals.
- Seven-point subjective global assessment score (SGA)
- Malnutrition inflammation score (MIS)
- Three-day dietary intake recall
- Anthropometry:
    - BMI/waist circumference
    - Skin fold thickness at the triceps or subscapular area
    - Mid-arm circumference
- Dual energy X-ray absorptiometry (DEXA)
- Biochemical markers
    - Plasma albumin concentration
    - Plasma transferrin
    - Plasma prealbumin and retinol-binding protein levels
- Multi frequency bioelectrical impedance analysis (MF-BIA)

MEDICAL NUTRITION THERAPY (MNT)

Medical nutrition therapy in CKD patients is tailor made to meet individual needs-based on nutritional status and comorbid conditions. The nutritional requirements keep on changing as kidney disease progresses and hence it is important to assess and revise the nutrition advise at regular intervals. Dietary counseling remains the mainstay of treatment for malnutrition.

A balanced diet for CKD patients depends on multiple factors:
- The stage of the disease
- If on dialysis, type of dialysis chosen (hemodialysis or peritoneal dialysis)
- Other co-morbidity (presence of diabetes/hypertension or other diseases)
- Height and weight
- Activity level
- Gastric problems
- Infections
- Urine output

Proteins

Dialysis is life-saving for many. However, the process is not as smart as the original kidney. Dietary proteins are usually restricted to 0.6–0.8 gm/kg/day in CKD patients not on dialysis to prevent net accumulation of acids, phosphorous and uric acid.

During dialysis, the body loses a portion of protein, vitamins, and minerals along with unwanted toxins, fluid, and chemicals. Hence it is important to switch to a high protein diet when a patient is initiated on dialysis.

As per kidney disease outcomes quality initiative (KDOQI) recommendation:
- Protein of 1–1.2 gm/kg/day for hemodialysis patients and 1.2–1.3 gm/kg/day for peritoneal dialysis patients is recommended.
- Minimum 65–70% of the protein should be from high biological value protein.
- **Animal sources of protein:** Meat, eggs, chicken, milk, seafood and cheese
- **Plant sources:** Nuts, seeds, legumes, pulses, soya and tofu

Calories

Patients on dialysis need ample energy to fight the diseases better. As per KDOQI an intake of 30–35 kcal per kg body weight per day is considered sufficient.
- **Fat:** Approx 25–30% of total calories should be from Fats.
- **Carbohydrates:** Minimum 60–65% of total calories should be through carbohydrates. Complex carbohydrates should be supplied in optimal levels to maintain calorie goals.

The recommended dietary requirements for different stages of CKD are shown in **Table 1**.

Major Electrolytes

Apart from Protein and calories there are three other major electrolytes to focus on a dialysis diet, i.e., sodium, potassium and phosphorus.

1. **Sodium:** It is necessary for maintaining blood pressure and fluid balance in the body. Sodium retention leads to high blood pressure and water retention and swelling on face, legs and hands. Patients should be advised to limit any readymade/packaged snacks, canned vegetables, sauces, salad dressing, pickles (any type), instant soup, noodles, etc.
2. **Potassium:**
   - The most important function of potassium is to control the functioning of nerves and muscles. Excess potassium in the body can cause irregular heartbeats and cardiac arrest.
   - Most fruits and vegetables are a good source of potassium.
   - The list of fruits and vegetables which dialysis patient can have and should avoid is mentioned in **Table 2**.

Table 1: Stages of chronic kidney disease and changes in nutrient requirement.

CKD stages 2–4	• Energy 30–35 kcal/kg/d • 35 kcal in <60 years • 30 kcal >60 years • Diabetics <30 kcal/kg/d • Low protein 0.6–0. 0.8 g/kg/d • Phosphorus 800–1,000 mg • Calcium 1,000–1,500 mg/d • Sodium <2.4 g/d • Potassium 1 mEq/kg • Cholesterol <200 mg/d • Water soluble vitamins and minerals as per RDA
CKD stage 5/ESRD on conservative management	Protein 0.6 mg/kg/day Rest same as patients on HD
Patient on hemodialysis and peritoneal dialysis	• Protein 1.2 g/kg/d (at least 50% should be of high biological value) • Calories 35 kcal/kg/d (<60 years) • 30–35 kcal/kg/d (60 years or older) • Total fat 25%-35% of total energy intake • Saturated fat <7% • Sodium 80–100 mmol • Potassium <1 mmol/kg if elevated • Cholesterol <200 mg • Total fiber 20–30 g/d

Table 2: Fruits and vegetables list for dialysis patients.

Fruits can have	***Fruits to avoid***	***Vegetables can have***	***Vegetables to avoid***
Apple	Citrus fruits	Brinjal	Spinach
Strawberry	Banana	Capsicum	Tomatoes
Pineapple	Dates	Cabbage	Potatoes
Grapes	Kiwi	Bottle gourd	Beans
Cranberries	Avocado	White radish	Pumpkin
Guava	Coconut water	Onion	Broccoli
Papaya	Apricots	Lettuce	Beets

- There is a simple procedure of "Leaching" to remove excess potassium from vegetables. Peel the vegetables and soak in water for an hour. Cut them and again soak in water for 4–5 hours and drain them. Wash them with water and cook them in excess water and drain that water again.

3. **Phosphorus:**
   - Foods rich in phosphorus are dairy foods, chocolate, nuts, soya and whole grains like oats, whole wheat, bajra, jowar, etc., along with pulses and dals.
   - Since most foods rich in phosphorus are also protein rich people undergoing dialysis are often supplemented with phosphate binders like sevelamer or calcium acetate which prevent the absorption of phosphorus from food.

Fluids

- Patients on hemodialysis need to restrict the intake of fluids depending on the amount of urine output left. The target is to keep Intradialytic weight gain less than 1.2–1.5 kg.
- One way to reduce fluid intake is to reduce salt intake which in turn reduces thirst. Patient can also be advised to drink from small cups throughout the day.

SUGGESTED READING

1. Ikizler TA, Burrowes JD, Byham-Gray LD, Campbell LK, Carrero J-J, Chan W, et al. KDOQI Clinical Practice Guideline for Nutrition in CKD: 2020 Update. Am J Kidney Dis Off J Natl Kidney Found. 2020;76(3 Suppl 1):S1-107.
2. Saxena A. Nutritional problems in adult patients with chronic kidney disease. Clin Queries Nephrol. 2012;1(3):222-35.
3. MacLaughlin HL, Friedman AN, Ikizler TA. Nutrition in Kidney Disease: Core Curriculum 2022. Am J Kidney Dis. 2022;79(3):437-49.

Vaccination in Chronic Kidney Disease

29
CHAPTER

Atul Kumar Srivastava, Bhupesh Kumar Saini, Manish R Balwani

INTRODUCTION

Chronic kidney disease (CKD) is associated with alteration in the immune system, as a result, patients become more susceptible to various infections, malignancy, and cardiovascular disease. In developing countries, infections are a major cause of morbidity and mortality in these patients. Vaccines are an important tool in preventing infections. However, CKD patients remain under-vaccinated. Due to the vulnerability of CKD patients to infection, an effective vaccine strategy is required in these patients. Vaccination in this subset of patients can prevent many life-threatening infections.

The response to vaccination is generally lower in this group of patients as their ability to fight infections. The reasons for poor response to vaccination are multifactorial, e.g., age, comorbidities, previous infection, poor nutrition, vaccine type, dose, etc.

Vaccines are most effective when they are administered early in the course of kidney disease. The list of common vaccines in CKD is given in **Figure 1**.

COMMONLY ADMINISTERED VACCINES

Hepatitis B Vaccine

The hepatitis B vaccine should be administered to all CKD patients. The prevalence of hepatitis B infection in patients on hemodialysis is 7.6% in India. They should be given increased doses as compared to normal adults. Recombinant vaccines are recommended. They should be given four doses early in the course of illness at 0, 1, 2 and 6 months. The vaccine should be given intramuscularly in the deltoid region of both arms. Antibody titer against hepatitis B surface antigen should be assessed after 2–3 months of complete vaccination. If a patient fails to mount

Vaccine	Age	Dose	Vaccination schedule/ route of administration
Hepatitis B, Engerix B®	≥20 years	40 mcg	0, 1, 2, and 6 months/IM
	<20 years	10 mcg	0, 1, and 6 months/IM
Pneumococcal	....	....	........Refer Table 13........
Influenza	3–8 years	15 µg	Each year/IM
	9–12 years	15 µg	Each year/IM
	>12 years	15 µg	Each year/IM
Varicella	1–12 years	0.5 mL	One single dose/SC
Hepatitis A, havrix®	>17 years	1440 U	0, 6–12 months/IM
Measles, mumps, and rubella	>18 years	0.5 mL	One single dose/SC
Inactivated poliovirus	<18 years	0.5 mL	Three doses with an interval of 1–2 months
Diphtheria and tetanus toxoids	7 years	0.5 mL	Three doses/IM

IM: Intramuscular, SC: Subcutaneous

Fig. 1: Vaccination in chronic kidney diseases.

an effective response to the vaccine, doses should be repeated. If a patient fails to take complete doses, vaccination should be repeated. Booster doses should be given if the anti-HBs level falls below 10 IU/mL.

Pneumococcal Vaccine

Pneumonia is an important cause of morbidity and mortality in patients with chronic kidney disease. All patients should receive pneumonia conjugate vaccine 13 (PCV 13) 0.5 mL intramuscularly in the deltoid region followed by pneumococcal polysaccharide vaccine 23 (PPSV 23) after 8 weeks. Both vaccines are sufficiently immunogenic in patients on dialysis. PPSV 23 efficacy wanes with time, PPSV can be repeated after 5 years. If the patient had received PPSV 23 as an initial vaccine, PCV 13 can be given after 1 year.

Influenza Vaccine

Influenza vaccines are recommended annually. They should be given before the beginning of the winter season in these patients. Household contacts should also be vaccinated with influenza vaccines to prevent transmission to CKD patients. Despite poor response in CKD patients, the vaccine remains effective in preventing serious flu infection. Patients on dialysis are vaccinated more commonly than nondialysis patients as these vaccines are administered as per protocol in various dialysis centers. Higher doses of vaccines have been found to provide better protection in solid organ transplant patients, hence the same strategy can be used in CKD patients. 0.5 mL of vaccine should be given intramuscularly in the deltoid region.

Measles, Mumps, and Rubella (MMR) Vaccines

MMR vaccines are recommended in all patients prior to kidney transplant. Outbreaks of measles, mumps, and rubella continue to occur worldwide. MMR vaccine should be given at least 4 weeks prior to transplant so that sufficient response could be obtained. Response to the vaccines varies for the three illnesses in all patients. MMR vaccine being a live vaccine, is contraindicated in kidney transplant recipients.

Diphtheria, Pertussis and Tetanus (DPT) Vaccine

The tetanus vaccine has poor immunogenicity in patients with CKD and in patients on dialysis. Kidney transplant patients achieve good seroconversion if vaccinated with the DPT vaccine after 4 weeks.

Varicella Vaccines

CKD patients who are nonimmune to varicella have a high risk of infection postkidney transplant. All patients on dialysis should be vaccinated within 2 years after starting dialysis and at least 4 weeks prior to kidney transplant. All patients should receive 2 doses of vaccine 4 weeks apart.

Hepatitis A Vaccine

The hepatitis A vaccine should be administered to all patients who are at risk. Immune response varies from person to person; hence two doses of vaccine should be given. Serology should be done to check for adequate immune response.

COVID-19 Vaccine

Two Covid-19 vaccines are available for use in India; the Oxford–AstraZeneca vaccine (ChAdOx1 nCov-19; Covishield) and BBV152 (Covaxin). Two doses of these vaccines are administered 4 weeks apart. Both these vaccines provide sufficient immunogenicity in CKD patients as well as kidney transplant patients. In patients on dialysis who are planning for a kidney transplant, vaccination should be done before the transplant.

Other Vaccines

Hemophilus influenza type B (HIB) conjugate vaccine should be given to all pediatric patients of CKD and the dose is similar to adults.

Staphylococcus aureus infections are common in patients with CKD. However, the response to the staphylococcal vaccine is less in patients with CKD. The immunological response wanes faster by 6 months (reduces by 50%). Due to limited data on efficacy, currently, this vaccine is not recommended.

Conclusion

CKD being an immunocompromised state exposes the patient to the risk of various life-threatening infections. However, with the available vaccines, morbidity, and mortality can be significantly reduced in these patients. Higher doses and increasing the frequency of vaccination may be required to get a sufficient immunogenic response in this subset of patients.

SUGGESTED READING

1. Guidelines for vaccination in patients with chronic kidney disease. Indian J Nephrol. 2016;26(Suppl 1):S15–8.
2. Haddiya I. Current Knowledge of Vaccinations in Chronic Kidney Disease Patients. Int J Nephrol Renovasc Dis. 2020;13:179-85.

Infection Control Measures and Biomedical Waste Disposal

Aslam Mohd, Shahbaj Zia Salari, Vivek Sood

INTRODUCTION

Hepatitis B and C, as well as other bloodstream infections, are common among dialysis patients. Hepatitis B and C are viral hepatitis transmitted via the bloodstream. B and C viruses may survive and transmit on surfaces without visible blood. When bacteria or other organisms enter the blood vessels, they cause a potentially severe disease known as a bloodstream infection. Germs may enter the bloodstream through a vascular access site, i.e., the catheter, graft, or fistula.

PREVENTION OF BLOOD STREAM INFECTIONS

"*Bloodstream infections*" are considered the most severe potential complications of dialysis. One in every four people with *Staphylococcus aureus* bloodstream infections has complications like:

- Endocarditis (heart valve disease)
- Osteomyelitis (bone infection)

What Causes Infections?

An infection requires three distinct conditions to develop:

1. Bacteria or viruses.
2. A germ-prone host.
3. A germ route from origin to host.

Germs travel from the source to the host via three modes of transmission: contact, droplet, and airborne transfer. Infections may spread during dialysis, usually via healthcare workers.

Prevention of Infections

Understand and implement infection control. Infection control is crucial for healthcare workers. Due to the increased infection risk, certain authorities issued advice for hemodialysis professionals.

- Maintain proper hand hygiene.
- Wear PPE
- Use safe injection techniques.

Hand Hygiene

When handling blood or other biological fluids, wash your hands with soap and water, as shown in **Figure 1**. Use an alcohol-based hand rub if your hands are not unclean. Good hand hygiene is one of the best strategies to fight infections.

- Before touching a patient
- Before injecting medication

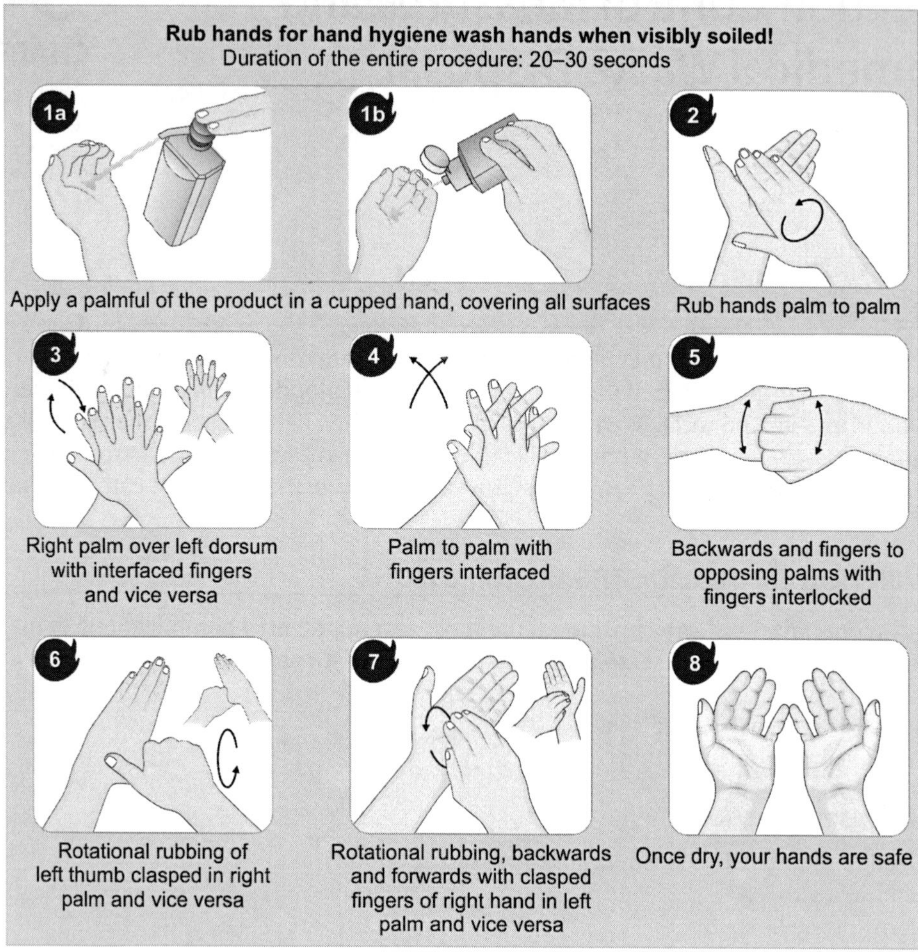

Fig. 1: Steps of hand washing and hygiene (as recommended by World Health Organization).

- Before cannulating a fistula/graft or accessing a catheter
- After touching a patient
- If you come into contact with blood, bodily fluids, mucosal membranes, wound dressing, or dialysis fluids
- Remove gloves after contacting dialysis station equipment.

Ensure Proper Use of PPE

- If you suspect you've touched blood or other infectious materials, use gloves, a gown, and/or face protection.
- Change gloves after touching an infected body part during medical treatment.
- Remove gloves after handling a patient or other infectious item.
- Do not reuse gloves on multiple patients.

Adhere to Safe Injection Procedures

Drugs are injected into the patient's bloodstream. The patient may become sick from medicine containers or syringe germs. A contaminated injection site might spread germs during the injection.

- Needles and syringes are single-use.
- Avoid giving many people IV or single-dose medicines.
- Before injecting, clean your hands and access the port.

Infection control protocols for hemodialysis professionals:

- Gloves and PPE must be used throughout patient care.
- Improve vascular access safety.
- Separate clean and contaminated spots.
- Handle medication vials with caution.
- Between patients, clean and disinfect the dialysis station.
- Safely handle dialysers.
- Wear gloves while cleaning near medical devices.
- Wash your hands after changing patients or dialysis stations.

INFECTION CONTROL IN FISTULA CARE

Cannulation Method

- Needles and syringes are single-use medical devices.
- Do not administer medicine to numerous patients at once from single-use vials or IV bags.
- Before administering an injection, practice good hand hygiene and cleanse the access port.

Decannulation Technique

- Maintain hand hygiene.
- Use a fresh pair of gloves.
- Wear appropriate facial protection.
- Remove needles aseptically.
- Use clean gauze/bandage for the affected area.
- Compress the place using clean gloves.

Catheter Connection Method

- Maintain hand hygiene.
- Wear clean gloves.
- Use facial protection.
- Clean the catheter hub with an antiseptic and let it dry.
- Aseptically attach the catheter to bloodlines. Release the catheter.
- Take off your gloves and clean your hands.

Catheter Disconnection Method

- Maintain hand hygiene.
- Use clean gloves.
- Use facial protection.

- Disconnect the catheter from the bloodlines aseptically.
- Antiseptically clean and dry the catheter hub.
- Aseptically replace caps.
- Keep the catheter clamped.
- Remove gloves and wash your hands.

OTHER INFECTION CONTROL MEASURES

Precautions for Catheter Exit Sites

- Maintain hand hygiene.
- Use clean gloves.
- Use facial protection.
- Disconnect the catheter from the bloodlines aseptically.
- Antiseptically clean and dry the catheter hub.
- Aseptically replace caps.
- Keep the catheter clamped.
- Remove gloves and wash your hands.

Supplies Designated for a Single Patient

- Anything brought to a patient's dialysis station may become infected.
- Do not return prescription bottles, syringes, or alcohol swabs to a clean communal area from the patient's unit.

Precautions for the Safe Use of Medication Vials

- Prepare patient doses in a sterile place away from dialysis stations.
- Prepare doses as soon as possible.
- Avoid transporting medical supplies between stations.
- Medication should not be prepared or stored at patient stations.

Carrying/Transporting Medications

- Do not share a medication cart.
- Avoid carrying vials, syringes, alcohol swabs, or other medical materials in your pockets.
- Safely prepare medication and bring it to the patient unit when needed.
- Cleaning and decontaminating the dialysis station reduces infection risk.

Do See

- Infection-causing germs on clean surfaces.
- Follow package instructions for dilution.
- Clean and disinfect using gloves.

Dialysis Station Decontamination

- After each patient treatment, disinfect the station.
- Clean all surfaces.

- Apply disinfectant and let dry.
- Clean and sanitize all waste containers.

Dialysis Machine and Blood Tubing Safety

Before removing or transferring dialysers, cap and clamp the blood tubing. Use leak-proof containers to transport used dialysers and tubing from the station to the reprocessing site.

Preventing the Spread of HBV/HCV/HIV

Patients who have HBV or HCV or HIV must be treated with dialysis in distinct rooms, utilizing separate machinery, apparatus, instruments, and supplies.

Prevent Bacterial Infections from Spreading

The following hemodialysis patients may spread germs to others:
- An infected, draining skin wound.
- Fecal incontinence or uncontrollable diarrhea.

Precautions When Treating these Patients

- Wear a gown and gloves while treating the patient, then take them off.
- Do not wear the same gown for many patients.
- If feasible, dialysis should be done in a corner or at the room's end.

BIOMEDICAL WASTE MANAGEMENT

Types of Hospital Waste (Table 1)

- Medical waste
- Biomedical waste
- Clinical waste
- Biohazardous waste
- Regulated medical waste (RMW)
- Infectious medical waste
- Healthcare waste
- Hospital waste

As per WHO, the following are the most prevalent waste categories. The types of waste and their categories are given in **Figure 2**.
1. **Sharps:** Needles, scalpels, lancets, shards of glass, razors, ampules, staples, wires, and trocars may penetrate human flesh.
2. **Infectious waste:** Swabs, tissues, excreta equipment, and lab cultures.
3. **Radioactive waste:** Discarded liquid from radiation or scientific inquiry and glassware and other items that have touched this liquid.
4. **Pathological waste:** Human fluids, tissue, blood, body pieces, physiological secretions, and infected animal corpses.
5. **Pharmaceuticals:** Unused, expired, or tainted drugs (antibiotics, injectables, and pills).
6. **Chemicals:** Mercury from damaged thermometers, disinfectants, laboratory solvents, batteries, and other medical equipment components.
7. **Genotoxic waste:** Cancerous, teratogenic, and mutagenic medical waste

Table 1: Different categories of waste with type of container and color coding.

Category	*Type of container*	*Color coding*
1. Human anatomical waste	Plastic bag	Yellow
2. Animal waste	Plastic bag	Yellow
3. Microbiology and biotechnology waste	Plastic bag	Yellow/red
4. Waste sharp	Puncture proof container	Blue/white
5. Discarded medicines and cytotoxic waste	Plastic bag	Black
6. Solid soiled waste	Plastic bag	Yellow/red
7. Solid waste (all disposable plastics)	Plastic bag	Blue
8. Liquid waste	Leak proof container	
9. Incineration waste	Plastic bag	Black
10. Chemical waste (solid)	Plastic bag	Black

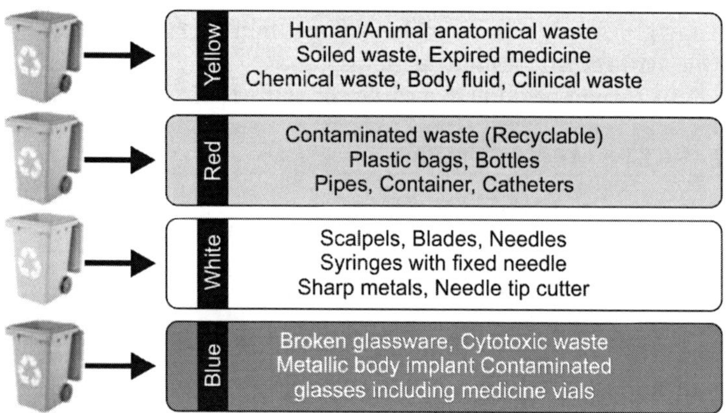

Fig. 2: Types of biomedical wastes and their color coding.

Steps for Managing Biomedical Waste

Step 1: Segregation: Segregation must be performed according to categories.

Step 2: Collecting and storage:

- **Location of the container:** All containers with colored polyethylene bags should be positioned at waste-producing sites near diagnostic services.
- **Bags:** Keep waste bags to a maximum capacity of 75%, knot them securely, and remove them from the source regularly.

  Storage of the waste:
  - No BMW should be kept untreated for more than 48 hours; if absolutely necessary, the authorized person must obtain permission from the appropriate authorities.
  - The authorized individual is responsible for ensuring that waste poses no threat to human health or the surroundings.

Step 3: Transportation:

- **Inside the hospital:**
  - To prevent mixing BMW with other trash, waste disposal channels should be developed, and a specific period defined for BMW.
  - Disinfect specialized wheeled carts after spills.
  - BMWs may only leave the hospital in government-approved cars.

Step 4: Treatment and disposal of waste:

- General trash accounts for 80–90% of hospital waste.
- It must be bagged in black polyethylene, disposed in municipal landfills, and collected by local authorities.

Biomedical Waste Management

- Disinfect and mutilate garbage before disposal.
- Deeply bury anatomical waste.
- Using hub cutters, syringes must be severed and chemically decontaminated at the generating source before disposal in a sharp's receptacle.

Incineration

"*BMW Rules 1998*" specifies combustion efficiency and emission levels:

- Install properly designed pollution control equipment.
- Incinerators need pollution control board approval.
- Avoid burning chlorinated plastic bags.
- No chlorinated disinfectants for burned garbage.
- CPCB rules require regular monitoring.
- Incinerator ash should be carried safely.

Burial

"BMW rule 1998" mandated corded deep burial for category one waste in rural regions under five lakh inhabitants. Floods and erosion should not occur.

- Autoclave and microwave
- **Needle destroyers:** Dispose of needles directly without using chemicals.
- **Shredding:** Plastic and sharps should be pulverized after chemical treatment, microwaving, and autoclaving.
- **Secured landfill:** Incinerator ash, wasted pharmaceuticals, cytotoxic chemicals, and solid chemical waste.

SUGGESTED READING

1. Karkar A. Infection control guidelines in hemodialysis facilities. Kidney Res Clin Pract. 2018;37(1):1-3. doi: 10.23876/j.krcp.2018.37.1.1. Epub 2018 Mar 31.
2. Karkar, Ayman; Bouhaha, Betty Mandin; Dammang, Mienalyn Lim. Infection Control in Hemodialysis Units: A Quick Access to Essential Elements. Saudi Journal of Kidney Diseases and Transplantation. 2014;25(3):496-19.
3. Prevention of Infection. Indian J Nephrol. 2020;30(Suppl 1):46-50.

Adequacy of Dialysis

31
CHAPTER

Sudeep Prakash, Aruna Acharya, RK Yadav

INTRODUCTION

The dialysis is initiated when it is assumed that kidneys are unable to carry out the excretory function for the body. This generally occurs when eGFR is less than 15 mL/min, along with presence of uremic signs and symptoms like nausea, vomiting, asthenia, anorexia, weight loss, intractable pruritus, inability to cope with daily routine, anemia, low serum albumin or low serum cholesterol.

The aim of dialysis is to relieve the patient of these signs and symptoms. When this goal is achieved, the dialysis is said to be adequate.

MEASURES OF DIALYSIS ADEQUACY

How does the technician decide, whether the parameters he has set for the patient's dialysis session are going to achieve the above goals or not. After all these will be achieved only after the patent has received 4–5 adequate dialysis sessions!

We have **Urea reduction rate (URR) and KT/v** to measure the adequacy of dialysis in each session.

Urea Reduction Ratio (URR)

URR tell about the percentage by which the serum urea is reduced. The formula is as follows: [{(Predialysis serum urea) – (postdialysis serum urea)}/Predialysis serum urea] × 100

Example 1: After a dialysis session postdialysis urea is 80 mg/dL and predialysis it was 200 mg/dL, URR will be

$$[(200-80)/200] \times 100 = 60\%$$

It should be measured every 12–14 treatments.

KT/V

Another method to measure dialysis adequacy is KT/v:

- **K stands for dialyser clearance:** Expressed in milliliters per minute (mL/min), it represents how much of the blood (in mL) has been cleared of its urea in each minute. It will vary with the blood flow through the dialyser (Kd). Please note that K_0A (Mass transfer area coefficient) is the maximum theoretical clearance that a dialyser can give for a given solute at infinite blood and dialysate flow rates.
- **t stands for time (in minutes):** Hence **Kt**, the numerator, is **clearly multiplied by time**. It thus stands for the volume of fluid completely cleared of urea during a that particular treatment.

V stands for **volume of distribution of urea**, which is equal to the volume of body water. There are many equations to calculate it, (e.g., Watson equation; Online mobile applications are available to calculate it. For example, https://www.qxmd.com/calculate/calculator_344) but for practical purpose it can be safely assumed to be 55–60% of postdialysis body weight. Thus KT/V is the volume passed through the dialyser in the entire session divided by the total volume in which urea is distributed, and **basically tells how many time the total volume (in which urea is distributed) has passed through the dialyser**.

KT/V is accurately calculated by **modified daugridas equation:**

$$\mathbf{Kt/V = -ln(R - 0.008 \times t) + (4 - 3.5 \times R) \times UF/W}$$

where ln is the natural logarithm, R is the ratio of postdialysis to predialysis serum urea, t is the session length (in hours), UF is the volume of fluid removed during dialysis (in liters), and W is the postdialysis weight **(here V has been assumed to be 55% of postdialysis body weight)**.

This may seem very complicated, but the use of mobile applications available for phones has made calculating this parameter very easy and practical. One such application is "Calculate by QxMD" **(Fig. 1)**. **KT/V can be directly calculated by Daugirdas equation using the following link** https://www.qxmd.com/calculate/calculator_128 and filling up Pre- and postdialysis urea, duration of dialysis, ultrafiltration, and postdialysis weight as is evident from the screenshot picture of the mobile application.

This application is also available on android play store and can also be downloaded through the following link: https://play.google.com/store/apps/details?id=com.qxmd.calculate.

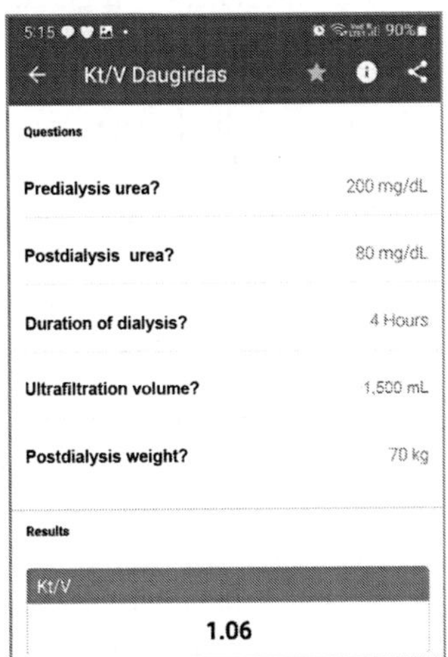

Fig. 1: Screenshot from the 'Calculate by Qx MD'.

Sampling of Urea

Predialysis urea sample should be taken during the placement of dialysis needles. For postdialysis sample there are two methods:

1. Slow the blood pump to 100 mL/min for 10–20 seconds. This will stop the backward blood flow returning needle to dialyser inlet needle. Thus, now all blood entering the arterial needle is upstream blood, and now the sample can be drawn from the sampling port.
2. Another way is to stop the dialysate flow for 3 minutes at the end of dialysis, and let the blood flow at the ongoing rate. After 3 minutes, the sample can be drawn from the sampling port.

URR vs KT/V

Though URR is easier to calculate, KT/V is more accurate as it takes clearance provided by ultrafiltration also into account. However, with the availability of mobile applications, KT/V has also become easily measurable. For the same URR if the UF is more the KT/V will be more in that session, where more UF was given. KT/V of 1.2 correlates to a URR of 63% (appox).

ADEQUATE DIALYSIS

Based on various data the kidney disease outcomes quality initiative (KDOQI) group recommends achieving a KT/V of at least 1.2 and URR 63–65%. Studies have shown that end stage kidney disease patients live longer, have better quality of life and have fewer hospitalizations if these targets are achieved. URR will be slightly below 65, if more UF is removed during dialysis. It is important to note that one odd KT/V <1.2 is not of concern, but it should be ensured that the average KT/V is 1.2. Various studies have shown that trying to achieve KT/V does not add to mortality benefit.

What measures should be taken to improve KT/V

KT/V should be measured every 12–14 dialysis sessions and if it is coming less than 1.2 consistently, then the nephrologist should review the dialysis parameters and take required action.

Following measures can be taken to improve KT/V:

- **Increase blood flow (Qb) through the dialyser (Fig. 2):** As discussed above, the K is actually Kd, which depends on the type of dialyser, and blood flow through it. As shown in the below figure, if the blood flow is low, then even with a large dialyser (high efficiency), the Kd delivered will not be much better than a low efficiency dialyser. However, the vascular access has to have good flow to achieve it.
- **Use a large dialyser:** As is evident from **Figure 1**, a dialyser with a larger surface area (high efficiency dialyser) will deliver a higher KT/V compared to a smaller surface area dialyser (low efficiency) at same Qb. In larger than average patients, two dialysers in series can also be used to increase the dialyser surface area.
- **Increase the dialyzate flow rate (Qd):** Good Qd is 2–3 times the Qb. A higher Qd ensures a higher concentration gradient for toxic nitrogenous waste, between blood and dialysate.
- Increase in 't' will increase the total clearance delivered (K in mL/min × duration of dialysis) in the session and hence will increase KT/V. For example, if Kd is 300 mL/min, t is 240 minutes (4 hrs), V is 50,000 mL (50 L), then KT/V= 1.44. If the t is increased to 300 minutes (5 hrs) the KT/V will increase to 1.88.
- Use the largest possible dialysis needle, to achieve good Qb. This depends on how well the vein downstream to AV fistula has matured. Needles from 14 G (largest) to 17 G (thinnest) are available.

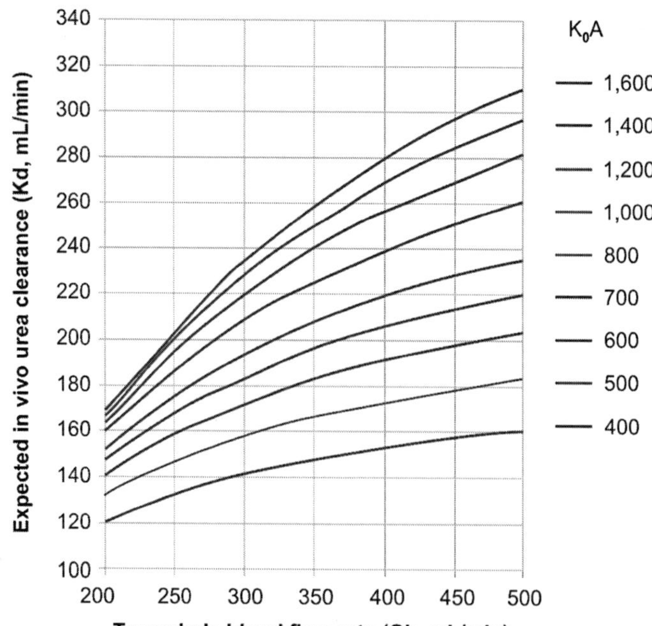

Fig. 2: Relationship between blood flow rate (QB) and dialyser blood water urea clearance (K) as a function of dialyser efficiency (K_0A). As the blood flow increases, the Kd increases.[1]

- **Increase the number of dialysis sessions per week:** This will increase the weekly KT/V also called as standard KT/V (std KT/V) to desired value of 2.1, in spite of low KT/V for each session.
- **Identify recirculation and try to reduce it:** Recirculation means that the dialyzed blood is entering the dialysis machine again, and hence the clearance (Kd) reduces. During recirculation, the concentration of urea in the blood entering the dialyser reduces by 5%–40%. The amount of urea removed in the dialyser is proportional to the volume of blood cleared and dialyser inflow urea concentration. Since the concentration of urea in the blood coming to the dialyser has reduced, the amount of urea removed is reduced in spite of 'K' and 't' remaining the same (i.e., same dialyser, same blood flow). This can occur due to inflow stenosis, very close placement of dialysis needles (arterial and venous lines) to each other, needle reversal.

SUGGESTED READING

1. Calculate by QxMD. [Internet]. Cited: 18 Jun 2023. Available from: https://play.google.com/store/apps/details?id=com.qxmd.calculate.
2. Daugirdas JT. Physiologic Principles and Urea Kinetic Modeling. In: Daugirdas JT, Blake PG, Ing TS,(Eds). Handbook of Dialysis, 5th edition. Wolters Kluwer Health publishing; 2015.
3. Hemodialysis Dose and Adequacy. https://www.niddk.nih.gov/-/media/Files/Kidney-Disease/hemodialysis_dose_508.pdf.
4. National Kidney Foundation: K/DOQI clinical practice guidelines for hemodialysis adequacy, 2000. American Journal of Kidney Disease. 2001;37(suppl 1):S7-64.

Duties and Responsibilities of Dialysis Technician

32
CHAPTER

Kishore Kumar A, Himanshu Sharma, Sanjeev Nair

INTRODUCTION

The dialysis team includes **technicians**, doctors, nurses, dieticians, and patients. Dialysis technicians are in immediate contact with the patient and are involved in direct care of the patient. Technicians are in a position to learn and share important information about patients with the team, which can improve care. Technicians should counsel patients and encourage them to participate actively in their care, improving their well-being and quality of life.

Dialysis technicians should strive to provide high-quality care to the patients, which should be:

- **Safe:** Making the dialysis process safer for the patient and minimizing the risks.
- **Timely:** To avoid delay in the care, which can be harmful to the patient sometimes.
- **Efficient:** To minimize wastage of supplies and equipment.
- **Effective:** Care should be effective-based on standard protocols.
- **Patient-centered:** Needs, wishes, and values of the patient are to be respected and addressed.
- **Equitable:** No discrimination-based on gender, income, education level, residence, and any other social category.

DUTIES AND RESPONSIBILITIES

Primary Duties

There are several duties and responsibilities of dialysis technicians which help in running the dialysis unit without quality or safety issues. They include:

- Technicians should check the water quality daily and keep a record. Dialysis should not be started until the water quality check is completed.
- Technicians should ensure the correct dialysate is delivered and ensure solutions are prepared correctly according to the established protocols.
- Predialysis evaluation of the patient should be done, which includes weight, pulse, blood pressure, temperature, respiration, physical state, swelling (edema), dialysis access (fistula or dialysis catheter) status, and problems since the last treatment.
- Check the patient's fistula before each session and ensure no problems. The exit site should be checked every time for patients with dialysis catheters to identify any infection.
- Avoiding infection in the dialysis unit and cross-spreading infection between the patients is essential. Washing hands before touching any fistula is the first step. Gloves used for one patient should not be used on another patient. Touch the fistula area and machines only with gloves on. Clean the skin of the fistula before needle insertion to avoid infection.
- The technician should calculate the amount of fluid removed-based on the patient's target dry weight and current weight. Saline rinses, priming saline, medications, and oral intake during the treatment should be included in the fluid removal planned during the session.

- Documentation of treatment provided, including the blood flow, dialysate flow, ultrafiltration, dialyser type, heparin dose used, weight of the patient before and after dialysis, pulse rate, blood pressure, complications during the procedure, treatment which is given, injections dose and route of administration is essential. Documentation helps in diagnosis, tracking, research, and as a legal document in case of a medicolegal issue.
- Alarms in the dialysis machine are to be addressed immediately and promptly to prevent danger to the patient's life. Knowing the meaning of each alarm type and learning the skill to manage the problem is vital in delivering dialysis care.
- The technician must check that dialysate lines are free from disinfectants. It is essential to check whether conductivity, pH, and dialysate temperature are within acceptable limits.
- In the case of a new dialyser, checks should be made for manufacturing defects and whether it is the same one prescribed by the nephrologist.
- In the case of dialyser reuse, the procedure for dialyser reuse should be strictly followed according to the dialysis unit policy. Checking the label during reuse for correct identification is very important, and make sure the disinfectant is rinsed off to avoid complications for the patient.

Supportive Duties

Technicians can help patients and doctors in a variety of ways:

- You can help in reducing the risk of anemia by preventing the dialyser from clotting, avoiding loss of blood while inserting and removing the needle, returning most of the blood to the patient after the dialysis session, reporting any unusual bleeding to the doctor and making sure patient completes the dialysis session full time.
- You can help provide an adequate dialysis dose by following the prescription given by the nephrologist.
- You can help in the medical management of the patient by asking the patient whether they are taking their medications appropriately.
- You can counsel the patient to follow diet and fluid limits. Reinforcing the boundaries multiple times can help better manage their diet. Technicians should Inform dieticians and doctors about patients who cannot follow the limits.
- You can help preserve the fistula (lifeline to the patient) by following good techniques during the insertion and removal of needles and by informing the problems with the fistula to the doctor immediately so that they can be addressed.

Additional Duties

One of the critical responsibilities of the technician is to be professional in their behavior which can be in many forms.

- Be on time to work and ready to work immediately.
- Wear clothes as guided by the administration of the dialysis unit.
- Please introduce yourself and your team to the patient and address them with their titles.
- Treat patients and their family members with respect and courtesy.
- Make sure all the equipment is ready and in working condition before the patient arrives.
- The patient care area should be kept clean, and the bed should be clean without any blood from previous treatment sessions.
- Do not shout, run or be noisy in the treatment area.
- Avoid discussing your personal life with a patient and in the dialysis unit.

- Protect the privacy of the patient and their confidential information.
- Avoid accepting money or gifts from patients or discussing personal problems with them.
- Never touch a patient inappropriately.
- Avoid giving advice and opining on the patient's personal problems. Do not get emotionally involved in their personal lives.

Technicians are the core members of the dialysis team who can bridge the gap between doctors and patients. Technicians should strive to make the dialysis procedure effective and safe, which helps in patient well-being.

SUGGESTED READING

1. Operational Guidelines for Dialysis Programme. Ministry oh Health and Family Welfare, Government of India. 2016.
2. Setting up of Hemodialysis Unit. Indian J Nephrol. 2020;30(Suppl 1):S1–S5.

Psychological Issues for Dialysis Patients

Shaurya Kaul, Amra Ahsan, Narinder Pal Singh

INTRODUCTION

Chronic kidney disease (CKD) is a widespread global health concern, affecting more than half of end-stage kidney disease (ESKD) patients undergoing dialysis. Hemodialysis, a common treatment for CKD, introduces its own set of issues, particularly in terms of mental and psychological well-being. Individuals grappling with CKD often contend with psychological challenges such as diminished self-esteem, heightened stress levels, depression, fear, anxiety, and emotional fluctuation making the management of their condition even more complex. Unfortunately, the psychological aspects of CKD care frequently go unnoticed by healthcare professionals, including attending doctors, technicians, and nurses. Additionally, the prescribed nonpsychiatric medications may not effectively alleviate the emotional distress symptoms experienced by these patients. Recognizing the pivotal role healthcare professionals play in the care and treatment of dialysis patients, it becomes crucial for them to not only focus on the technical aspects but also comprehend and address the psychological hurdles faced by these individuals. This chapter seeks to enlighten dialysis technicians about the psychological issues prevalent among dialysis patients and proposes strategies for tackling these challenges with empathy and comprehensive care.

THE PSYCHOLOGICAL IMPACT OF CHRONIC ILLNESS (FIG. 1)

- **Depression and anxiety:** The persistent nature of kidney disease and the rigorous demands of dialysis can lead to heightened feelings of depression and anxiety. These emotional challenges have a substantial impact on the well-being of both hemodialysis patients and their caregivers, influencing various aspects of their lives, including social, economic, and psychological dimensions. Indications of depression encompass feelings of sadness, anxiety, reduced self-confidence, a pessimistic outlook, diminished libido, disruptions in sleep patterns, and loss of appetite. It is crucial for technicians to be attentive to these signs and symptoms, collaborating closely with healthcare professionals to address mental health issues effectively.
- **The primary source of stressors for CKD:** The primary sources of stress for individuals dealing with CKD encompass financial challenges, alterations in social and marital relationships, frequent hospital admissions, restricted mobility, concerns about disability or mortality, heightened reliance on artificial renal machines, uncertainties about the future, and physical fatigue, with the most prevalent factors being. These stressors have the potential to induce both psychological and physical strain, often stemming from lifestyle modifications or adjustments in daily habits prompted by the condition.
- **Grief and loss:** Patients may experience a sense of loss related to their health, normal daily routine, lifestyle, uncertainty about the future, loss of self-esteem, independence, and financial strain. Understanding the stages of grief can aid technicians in providing empathetic support during difficult times.

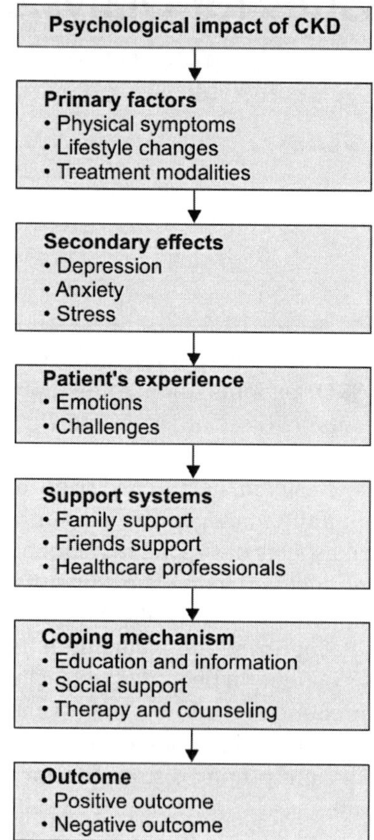

Fig. 1: Psychological impact of CKD and its coping strategies.

- **Effect of CKD on quality of life:** The quality of life (QoL) for individuals with CKD and their families is intricately connected to alterations in lifestyle and daily routines. At the same time, the well-being of CKD patients is profoundly influenced in terms of physical health, functional capabilities, personal relationships, and socio-economic status. Studies emphasize that factors such as reduced kidney function, fatigue, and disruptions in sleep patterns play pivotal roles in diminishing QoL. Mental health issues are notably prevalent among those with chronic renal failure, given the heightened levels of stress, social isolation, and fatigue they often experience. Regrettably, there is a common shortfall in doctors' knowledge of psychiatric disorders, leading to a lack of proper attention to these issues when patients require it.
- **Energy:** Energy constitutes a fundamental aspect of overall well-being, and for individuals with CKD, maintaining sufficient energy levels for various activities, from work to recreation, can be particularly challenging. Chronic kidney disease often contributes to persistent feelings of low energy, fatigue, and a pale appearance in patients. Fatigue, a significant stressor, can profoundly impact a person's ability to engage in work and various activities, and it may be exacerbated by sleep disorders or exhaustion following hemodialysis. The resulting physical or mental fatigue has a notable impact on the lives of individuals with CKD.

- **Impact on family life:** The presence of a loved one with CKD has a profound impact on families, giving rise to a spectrum of emotions and specific needs. Coping with a chronic illness poses challenges for both families and caregivers, treating CKD as a medical crisis within the family dynamic. For families, the changes in the personality of individuals with CKD undergoing hemodialysis can prove to be more challenging to endure than the physical limitations they may face. Despite advancements in patient survival, the care of individuals with chronic renal disease and earlier stages of CKD continues to impose substantial psychosocial, emotional, and economic stress on families.
- **Personality factor:** Patients with CKD commonly experience challenges in their personal and emotional responses. Survivors of CKD may exhibit altered behaviors, expressing emotions such as anger, anxiety, and caution that are markedly different from their usual personalities. This can lead the individual to feel victimized and perceive a diminished sense of self. While research on personality dysfunctions in CKD is limited, a study by Koutsopoulou et al. regarding the impact of chronic hemodialysis on patients' personalities revealed that those undergoing dialysis often display significant psychological personality disorders, including alexithymia, neuroticism, introversion, and psychoticism.
- **Self-care:** Patients with chronic kidney disease may encounter difficulties in performing routine daily activities due to factors such as fatigue. Tasks that were once part of their regular activities, like exercise and self-care, may become challenging. The perception of the disease can significantly impact the mental health of patients, influencing disease management and shaping their approach to self-care behavior.
- **Social role:** The physical and psychological impacts of CKD can result in notable shifts in the survivor's social standing. Nearly two-thirds of respondents acknowledged that their families and social lives were somehow affected. This effect is particularly pronounced in patients whose mobility is severely limited due to disabilities. Certain survivors perceive that their circumstances have eroded their relationships and curtailed their participation in broader social activities, contributing to feelings of social isolation. In an effort to avert physical disabilities, some individuals have taken measures such as relocating or ceasing activities like driving.

STRATEGIES FOR TACKLING THE PSYCHOLOGICAL CHALLENGES IN CKD

Coping Mechanisms

- **Education and information:** Providing patients with clear and understandable information about their condition and treatment can empower them and reduce anxiety. Technicians should be prepared to answer questions and offer educational resources.
- **Support systems:** Encouraging patients to build a support network can alleviate feelings of isolation. Technicians can facilitate connections with support groups or counseling services.
- **Mind-body techniques:** Mindfulness and meditation/deep breathing exercises can help reduce anxiety and improve mental well-being.
- **Adaptive problem solving:** Breaking down larger challenges into smaller, manageable goals can make the journey more achievable. Actively problem-solving and seeking solutions to challenges can empower patients and reduce feelings of helplessness.

Communication Skills

- **Active listening:** Developing strong communication skills, particularly active listening, helps technicians understand patients' concerns and emotions. Acknowledging and validating patients' feelings can enhance the therapeutic relationship.

- **Empathy and compassion:** Expressing empathy and compassion fosters trust and emotional well-being. Technicians should be mindful of the impact their words and actions can have on the emotional state of patients.

Addressing Fear and Uncertainty

- **Transparent communication:** Openly discussing treatment plans, potential complications, and expectations can reduce uncertainty. Technicians should be prepared to address fears and concerns, providing reassurance where possible.
- **Routine and predictability:** Establishing a predictable routine in the dialysis setting can offer a sense of control for patients. Technicians can contribute to this by maintaining consistent practices and schedules.

Recognizing Warning Signs

- **Suicidal ideation:** Dialysis patients may be at an increased risk of suicidal thoughts. Technicians should be trained to recognize warning signs and report concerns promptly to the healthcare team.
- **Severe anxiety or panic attacks:** Some patients may experience severe anxiety or panic attacks during dialysis sessions. Technicians should be equipped to respond calmly, following established protocols.

CONCLUSION

Understanding the psychological challenges encountered by individuals undergoing dialysis is essential for delivering comprehensive care. Patient compliance with chronic disease management is notably shaped by the support they receive from their social or family network, along with the assistance provided by medical staff. Dialysis technicians, positioned uniquely in patient care, can play a pivotal role in promoting the emotional well-being of those undergoing dialysis. When facing a chronic health issue, individuals with robust support systems often employ adaptive strategies to cope with the disease. Healthcare professionals, through effective communication, empathy, and creating a supportive environment, play a crucial role in guiding patients through the psychological dimensions of their health journey. Ongoing education and training in this domain contribute to enhancing the overall quality of care delivered by dialysis teams.

SUGGESTED READING

1. Alkhaqani AL. Psychological Impact of Chronic Kidney Disease and Hemodialysis: Narrative Review. Psychosom Med Res. 2022;4(2):3. doi: 10.53388/202209.
2. Cukor D, Cohen SD, Peterson RA, Kimmel PL. Psychosocial aspects of chronic disease: ESRD as a paradigmatic illness. J Am Soc Nephrol. 2007;18(12):3042-55.
3. Gerogianni SK, Babatsikou FP. Psychological aspects in chronic renal failure. Health Sci J. 2014;8(2):205-14.
4. Koutsopoulou-Sofikiti EB, Kelesi-Stavropoulou NM, Vlachou DE, Fasoi-Barka GG. The effect of chronic dialysis in personality of patients with chronic renal failure. Vima Asklipiou. 2009;8(3):240-54.

End-of-Life Care and Withholding Dialysis

34
CHAPTER

Anish Kumar Gupta, Gurleen Kaur, Narinder Pal Singh

INTRODUCTION

Caring for our loved ones as they approach the end of their lives involves a complex mix of psychological, medical, emotional, spiritual, ethical, cultural, ethnic, legal, and familial factors. Healthcare professionals are faced with the challenge of reevaluating current approaches to end-of-life care discussions. When it comes to providing end-of-life care for individuals on dialysis, there are several crucial elements, such as advance directives, dialysis withdrawal, do not resuscitate orders (DNR), palliative care, and hospice.

These aspects need careful attention at different stages of the assessment and treatment processes, involving both patients and their caregivers. Unfortunately, many dialysis technicians often overlook or neglect these critical components. This oversight can lead to problematic and distressing situations for patients and their families, situations that might be preventable. Dialysis professionals have also expressed concerns about the insufficient provision of quality care, citing unaddressed requirements such as the absence of discussions on end-of-life care and inadequate bereavement support.

This chapter outlines the end-of-life care process and identifies indicators of a dismal prognosis among dialysis patients, emphasizing the growing focus on this aspect of care. It elucidates the factors influencing the decision to continue dialysis despite an unfavorable prognosis. The final section underscores the importance of shared decision-making in the judicious initiation and withholding of dialysis.

END-OF-LIFE CARE

Patients with CKD often lack understanding of palliative and hospice care, nephrology providers seldom discuss end-of-life care preferences with patients, and many renal care units feel unprepared for such discussions due to inadequate training. To provide adequate end-of-life care, discussions on patient preferences and goal documentation are essential. Advance care planning (ACP) tools based on patient perspectives aim to facilitate these discussions. Early ACP in CKD, legally documented, ensures care aligns with patients' wishes, crucial for patients with cognitive impairment. Communication about the option to discontinue dialysis is vital, with hospice services recommended for managing symptoms and providing support in these cases.

Factors Indicating Increasing Attention to End-of-Life Care

The emergence of palliative medicine as a specialized field within healthcare plays crucial roles in elevating awareness regarding palliative care, as well as decisions involving withdrawing from or withholding dialysis. Presently, a universally accepted set of criteria for refraining from dialysis is lacking. Several factors contribute to the growing emphasis on end-of-life care for individuals dealing with ESRD. Predictors for poor prognosis among dialysis patients involve:

- Senior citizens (as per research designating adverse results for individuals aged 75 years and above);
- Individuals with elevated comorbidity indices (e.g., modified Charlson Comorbidity Index score of 8 or higher);
- Significant functional limitations (e.g., Karnofsky Performance Status Scale score below 40)
- Intense chronic malnutrition (e.g., serum albumin level below 2.5 g/dL)

Individuals in this population should be made aware that opting for dialysis might not necessarily result in enhanced survival or improved functional status when compared to medical management without dialysis. Additionally, undergoing dialysis carries substantial burdens that could impact their overall quality of life.

Factors that may Contribute to Ongoing Dialysis Despite Dismal Prognosis

Despite advancements in palliative care and dismal prognosis emotional challenges persist in dialysis programs, marked by terms like "torture" and "dialyzing the dead." To address these issues, it's crucial to examine factors contributing to continued dialysis in the face of a grim prognosis include:

- **Patient-related factors** encompass diverse aspects such as goals, values, demographics, religious beliefs, decision-making capacity, and the absence of a designated decision maker.
- **Physician-related challenges** include discomfort with end-of-life discussions, legal fears, religious considerations, and the consultative nature of nephrology.
- **System-related issues** involve legal statutes, deficient advance care planning, transitions of care, time constraints for planning, and insufficient training in communication and palliative care.

Addressing these multifaceted factors is vital to navigating the complexities of end-of-life decisions in dialysis programs.

Recommendation on Shared Decision-making in the Appropriate Initiation of and Withholding from Dialysis

- Encouraging shared decision-making is advised for the patient-healthcare professional relationship in all cases of ESRD.
- For patients with ESRD, choices in shared decision-making encompass:
  - Various available dialysis modalities and, when relevant, kidney transplantation
  - Opting not to initiate dialysis and instead continuing with medical management
  - A time-limited trial of dialysis: In cases of uncertain prognosis or when consensus on providing dialysis is elusive, nephrologists may contemplate proposing a time-limited trial of dialysis for patients in need
  - Stopping dialysis and receiving end-of-life care.
- **Making a decision to withhold dialysis:** If deemed appropriate, abstain from initiating or cease ongoing dialysis for ESRD patients in specific, well-defined situations. These include instances where patients with decision-making capacity voluntarily decline or request discontinuation. Additionally, this applies to patients without decision-making capacity who previously expressed refusal in an advance directive or, in their absence, when appointed legal agents/surrogates decline or request discontinuation. Furthermore, patients with irreversible, profound neurological impairment lacking signs of cognition or awareness are also included in these considerations.
- Patients, or their legally designated representatives in case of decision-making challenges, should be empowered to make choices among available options. This includes the autonomy

to decide between passing away in a healthcare facility or opting for hospice care at home. Furthermore, families of patients should receive necessary bereavement support.

- Fully inform patients about their diagnosis, estimating prognosis, and all treatment options.
- Their decisions should be informed and voluntary.
- Conversations regarding life expectancy and quality of life should occur with the patient or their legal representative. It is suitable to engage in discussions and potentially reevaluate treatment objectives, including the consideration of withholding dialysis.
- **Conflict resolution:** Resolving conflicts about the benefits of dialysis requires a systematic approach. This is essential when disagreements arise between the patient or their legal representative and the renal care team. Conflicts may also emerge within the renal care team or with other healthcare providers. The resolution process should examine potential sources of conflict, such as miscommunication about prognosis, interpersonal issues, or differing values. Urgently needed dialysis should proceed during conflict resolution if requested by the patient or legal representative.
- The renal care team, working collaboratively with the primary care physician, must guarantee that the patient or authorized representative comprehends the advantages and drawbacks of dialysis and the repercussions associated with either commencing or discontinuing dialysis.
- Likewise, evidence-based recommendations assist renal care team members in effectively informing and advising patients and families regarding possible outcomes of ESRD.
- **Providing effective palliative care in CKD:** Palliative care for ESRD adopts a comprehensive strategy, emphasizing comfort and assistance for patients and their families facing chronic or terminal illnesses. This all-encompassing approach tackles physical symptoms while acknowledging the emotional and spiritual aspects of distress. Key elements encompass well-defined procedures for pain control, proactive planning for future care, facilitating hospice referrals for those opting to discontinue dialysis, offering psychosocial and spiritual assistance, and implementing bereavement initiatives. Dialysis units incorporate renal palliative care principles into their policies, complying with coverage requirements and quality care evaluations.
- Because everyone is different, they have unique values and goals. This means some people might choose treatments or ongoing care that others wouldn't. To be ethical and provide the best care, it's important to give patients and their families all the information they need. This helps them make decisions together with the healthcare team. By doing this, we make sure everyone involved—patients, families, and healthcare providers in dialysis—feels satisfied with the care choices made.
- **Advance directives:** The renal care team should make efforts to acquire written advance directives from every dialysis patient, and these directives must be respected and followed.
- **Ethical principles:** The embrace of shared decision-making, aligned with core ethical principles like autonomy, beneficence, nonmaleficence, and distributive justice, establishes the discontinuation of dialysis as both ethically sound and clinically justifiable.

CONCLUSION

End-of-life care provided by the renal care unit involves compassionate support for patients undergoing dialysis as they approach the final stages of life. Healthcare professionals play a crucial role in ensuring patients' comfort, dignity, and emotional well-being during this challenging time. They may collaborate with multidisciplinary healthcare teams to address patients' specific needs, facilitate open communication about treatment options, and assist in the transition to palliative care or hospice services. Dialysis technicians contribute to maintaining a respectful and caring environment, emphasizing the importance of discussions around end-of-life preferences. Their involvement in this process underscores the holistic approach to patient care, acknowledging the unique challenges faced by individuals undergoing dialysis nearing the end of life.

SUGGESTED READING

1. Combs SA, Davison SN. Palliative and end-of-life care issues in chronic kidney disease. Curr Opin Support Palliat Care. 2015;9(1):14-9.
2. Galla JH. Clinical practice guideline on shared decision-making in the appropriate initiation of and withdrawal from dialysis. The Renal Physicians Association and the American Society of Nephrology. J Am Soc Nephrol. 2000;11(7):1340-42.
3. Jean LH. Palliative Care and Withholding and Withdrawing Dialysis. Dialysis & Transplantation 2011;40(4):154-5.

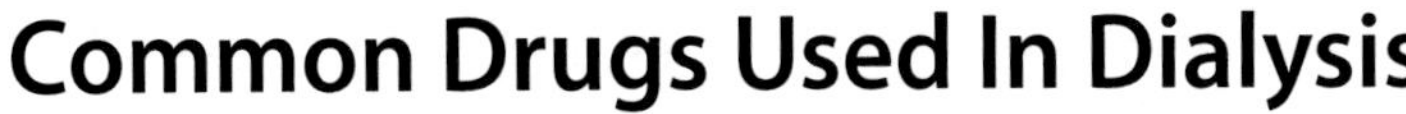

Common Drugs Used In Dialysis

Aslam Mohd, Shahbaj Zia Salari, Narinder Pal Singh

1. Adrenaline (epinephrine)	
Clinical use	Sympathomimetic and inotropic drug
Dose	0.01–1 mcg/kg/min
Route	IV, IM, S/C
2. Noradrenaline (norepinephrine)	
Clinical use	Hypotension, Vasopressor
Dose	Acute hypotension 40 mcg/mL, initially start with 0.16–0.33 mL/min Cardiac arrest 200 mcg/mL solution
Route	IV
3. Atropine	
Clinical use	Symptomatic bradycardia and inhibition of secretions
Dose	0.6–1.2 mg IV
Route	IV, IM, SUBQ
4. Ondansetron	
Clinical use	Anti emetic
Dose	Oral 4–32 mg daily in 2–3 divided doses IV 8–32 mg daily
Route	IV, IM, Oral, Rectal
5. Sodium bicarbonate	
Clinical use	Metabolic acidosis and urine alkalinization
Dose	Oral—500–1,000 mg BD-TDS IV—8.4%, 60–120 mL per hour
Route	Oral, IV
6. Potassium chloride	
Clinical use	Hypokalemia
Dose	Injection 10% KCL
Route	Oral, IV
7. Tramadol	
Clinical use	As analgesic
Dose	Oral—50–100 mg up to 4 hours (max. 400 mg daily) IM/IV- 50m-100 mg every 4–6 hourly (max. 400 mg/day)
Route	IV, IM, oral

8. Furosemide	
Clinical use	Loop diuretic
Dose	Oral—20 mg to 1 g daily IV—20 to 1.5 gm daily
Routes	IV, Oral
9. Chlorpheniramine	
Clinical use	Allergic reaction and dialyser reaction
Dose	Oral—75 mg once or twice IV/IM—1–2 mL (22.75 mg/mL)
Routes	IM, IV, Oral
10. Hydrocortisone	
Clinical use	Anaphylactic shock, Allergic reaction, Anti-inflammatory, and Others
Dose	Oral—20–30 mg in divided doses for replacement IV/IM—100–500 mg, 3–4 times in 24 hours or as required
Routes	Oral, IV, IM
11. Heparin	
Clinical use	Anticoagulant in dialysis
Dose	IV—loading dose of 5,000 IU, then continuous infusion 18 units/kg/hour SC—5,000 IU BD (dose to be adjusted as per eGFR)
Dialysis	5,000 IU stat followed 1,000 mg/hour
Route	IV infusion or bolus, SC
12. Epoetin Alfa	
Clinical use	Anemia of CKD (erythropoietin stimulating agents)
Dose	4,000–10,000 IU SC 2–3 times/week
Route	SC
13. Darbepoetin Alfa	
Clinical use	Anemia of CKD (erythropoietin stimulating agents)
Dose	25–40 mcg SC 1/week
Route	SC
14. Mircera	
Clinical use	Anemia of CKD (long acting erythropoietin stimulating agents)
Dose	50–100 mcg SC (once in 15 d – 30 days)
Route	SC
15. Dextrose	
Clinical use	Hypoglycemia
Dose	25–50 mL push over 3 minutes
Route	IV

16. Vancomycin	
Clinical use	Antibiotic (Antistaphylococcus)—CRBSI
Common dosing	500 mg–1,000 mg IV
Route	IV
17. Iron sucrose	
Clinical use	Iron supplementation in iron deficiency
Dose	100–200 mg during dialysis
Route	IV
18. Ferric carboxy maltose	
Clinical use	Iron supplementation in iron deficiency
Dose	500–1,000 mg
Route	IV
19. Calcium carbonate	
Clinical use	Phosphate binding agent Calcium supplement
Dose	500–1,000 mg BD-TDS
Route	Oral
20. Calcitriol	
Clinical use	Active vitamin D (renal osteodystrophy, CKD-MBD)
Dose	Oral—0.25 mcg daily or alternate day adjust dose by 0.25 mcg p/day
Route	Oral
21. Midodrine	
Clinical use	Hypotension
Dose	5 mg orally
Route	Oral
22. Labetalol	
Clinical use	Hypertensive crisis
Dose	Oral—50–400 mg twice daily, 20 mg IV bolus
Route	IV, oral
23. Nitroglycerine	
Clinical use	Hypertensive crisis
Dose	Vial 50 mg/10 mL, 0.25–0.5 mcg/kg/minute continuous IV infusion
Route	IV

Appendices

APPENDIX A: INFORMED CONSENT FOR HEMODIALYSIS (HD)

NAME		PHONE NO.		AGE/SEX	
ADDRESS					

Please read the content carefully. Do ask if you have any further questions. The doctors/staff members in this department are here to help you.

1. HD is necessary for patients whose kidneys are not functioning, either temporarily or permanently.
2. HD is a life-sustaining procedure, not a cure for kidney failure.
3. The procedure is necessary to treat my condition and has been explained to me by my physician.
4. Following risks are associated with HD
   a. Bacterial and/or viral (e.g., hepatitis B or C) contamination of my blood which may cause infection or bacterial infection of the blood called sepsis.
   b. Bleeding and coagulopathy associated with anticoagulation therapy.
   c. "Destruction" or the breakdown of red blood cells, known as hemolysis.
   d. Internal bleeding or bleeding from the access site.
   e. Infections of my access site (catheter or fistula infections)
   f. Introduction of air into my bloodstream
   g. Shock or cardiac arrest.
   h. Allergic and toxic reactions to drugs, solutions, dialysers, or other equipment used during the hemodialysis treatment.
   i. Clotting of my access.
   j. Technical/equipment malfunction and failure.
5. Though the above-said risks are not common, one or more can occur and be potentially life-threatening.
6. There may be some side effects associated with hemodialysis; they are osteoporosis, electrolyte imbalance, headache, nausea, dizziness, fainting, irregular heartbeats, decrease in blood pressure, decrease in urine output, muscle cramping, and mild confusion.
7. Other urgent procedures in addition to HD may be carried out as a life-saving or preventive measure.
8. Preliminary and periodic investigation and blood tests are required to assure safe and effective treatment, including screening for various communicable diseases such as CMV, hepatitis and HIV.

DECLARATION BY THE PATIENT
"I, ________________________ (name of patient/NOK) hereby declare that, I have read and fully understood the above points carefully/have been explained the above points in the language known by me with satisfactory answers to any questions that I have asked. I accept that there is a chance that the procedure might not be successful and no guarantees can be given as to the results. Understanding these limitations, I hereby give my informed consent to perform the hemodialysis therapy of my own free will."

Signature of Patient
Date:

Signature of NOK
Date:

Signature of Witness
Date:

APPENDIX B: CHECKLIST FOR DIALYSIS EXTERNAL DISINFECTION

Gather Supplies:

1. Personal protective equipment (PPE): eye goggles, gown, and clean gloves.
2. Properly diluted hospital disinfectant and wipes/cloths.
3. Biohazard disposal containers.

Perform:

4. Perform hand hygiene.
5. Don gown, eye goggles, and clean gloves.
6. Disconnect and take down used blood tubing and dialyser from the dialysis machine.
7. Check that there is no visible soil or blood on surfaces.
8. Ensure that the patient has left the dialysis station. Patients should not be removed until he/she is stable and if not, then delay routine disinfection.
9. Discard all single-use supplies. Move any reusable supplies.
10. Remove gloves and perform hand hygiene.

Disinfect Dialysis Station:

11. Perform hand hygiene and don clean gloves. Take a disinfectant-soaked wipe/cloth.
12. Using circular hand motion, disinfect all surfaces in the dialysis station including the dialysis bed, tray tables, blood pressure cuffs, etc. Clean dialysis machine from top to bottom. Clean the touch-screen monitor (activate the wipe screen option).
13. Clean the top of the machine. Clean exposed surfaces of dialysate, concentrate, and bicarb connectors.
14. Ensure surfaces are visibly wet with disinfectant but not dripping. Allow surfaces to air-dry.
15. Remove gloves, eye goggles, and gown. Perform hand hygiene.

APPENDIX C: STEPS FOR DIALYSIS MACHINE INTERNAL DISINFECTION

Gather Supplies:

1. Personal protective equipment (PPE): eye goggles, gown, and clean gloves.
2. Manufacturer-recommended disinfectant in required volume (most newer machines also have an additional filter, e.g., Diasafe or Diacap filters, for provision of ultrapure water/dialysate and use of disinfectants other than the manufacturer-recommended ones, may damage this filter).

Perform:

3. Don gown, eye goggles, and clean gloves.
4. Disconnect and take down used blood tubing and dialyser from the dialysis machine.
5. Ensure that the patient has left the dialysis station. Patients should not be removed until he/she is stable and if not, then delay routine disinfection.
6. Attach the dialyser and concentrate-line couplings to its attachment on the HD machine.
7. Bring the HD machine to the disinfection mode and select disinfection mode and disinfectant type.
8. Place the disinfectant line (may be variably located in front or back of the machine depending on the manufacturer) in the disinfectant container (not required if thermal disinfection is selected).
9. Begin disinfection and monitor it running.
10. At the end of chemical disinfection, remove the disinfectant container and test for residual disinfectant in outflow water. Continue in rinsing mode if residue is detected, till the indicator test is negative (skip this step for thermal disinfection and chemical disinfection with Citric Acid 50%).
11. Now, the HD machine is ready to be brought to HD mode and to receive another patient.

APPENDIX D: STEPS FOR BICARBONATE MIXER DISINFECTION

Gather Supplies:

1. Personal protective equipment (PPE): eye goggles, gown, and clean gloves.
2. Recommended disinfectant.

Perform:

3. Don gown, eye goggles, and clean gloves.
4. Discard any extra bicarbonate concentrate in the mixer.
5. Fill the mixing tank with a prespecified amount of RO water and then mix with either sodium hypochlorite (bleach) or commercial cleansing agents (the amount of solution must consider the volume of the tank as well as the total volume of the delivery loop). The solution should be kept in the mixer for a prespecified dwell time.
6. Then pump the solution to the head tank of the loop delivery system and ensure an even coating of the internal surface of the head tank through a spray nozzle.
7. After a specified dwell time, pump the solution through the delivery loop and check each patient station port for the presence of bleach or disinfectant to ensure delivery of disinfectant throughout the delivery loop.
8. Drain out the solution and rinse with RO water to remove bleach or disinfectant from the mixer, head tank, and delivery loop (till the test for residual disinfectant is negative at all patient station ports).
   - If delivery of bicarbonate solution through containers is being done then omit steps 6 onwards and to disinfect the containers, rinse them with RO water daily and with bleach solution once a week followed by RO water rinsing.
   - If bleach is being used for disinfection, then use acid rinse with acetic or citric acid once a week to remove carbonate deposition from the mixer, head tank, and delivery loop, in a fashion similar to the disinfection procedure (not required if a commercially available cleansing agent is used).

Index

Page numbers followed by *f* refer to figure and *t* refer to table.

A

B

C

D

I

J

K

L

M

N